ENT MCQs for Medical Students

with explanatory answers

GURDEEP SINGH MANNU
Foundation Year Doctor
Norfolk and Norwich University Hospital

AND

TUNDE ODUTOYE
Consultant ENT, Head and Neck Surgeon
St George's Hospital, University of London

Foreword by
SAMIR SOMA

Radcliffe Publishing
Oxford • New York

Radcliffe Publishing Ltd
18 Marcham Road
Abingdon
Oxon OX14 1AA
United Kingdom

www.radcliffe-oxford.com
Electronic catalogue and worldwide online ordering facility.

British Library Cataloguing in Publication Data

A catalogue record for this book is available from the British Library.

ISBN-13: 978 184619 389 7

The paper used for the text pages of this book
is FSC certified. FSC (The Forest Stewardship
Council) is an international network to promote
responsible management of the world's forests.

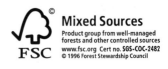

Mixed Sources
Product group from well-managed
forests and other controlled sources
www.fsc.org Cert no. SGS-COC-2482
© 1996 Forest Stewardship Council

Typeset by Pindar NZ, Auckland, New Zealand
Printed and bound by TJI Digital, Padstow, Cornwall, UK

Contents

Foreword

I was delighted to have the opportunity to write the foreword to this book. I met the co-author during his elective stint in South Africa, when I was fortunate enough to review this text. It presents a core knowledge of ENT in a self-test format with quick short answers so that the reader can review and identify those topics which require further reference.

Most textbooks intended for undergraduates are in a symptom-based format that allows the reader to grasp the scope of ENT quickly and easily. This knowledge is usually amassed in a two-week practical rotation, and is intended to equip an individual with the knowledge to manage 80% of GP visits. This, unfortunately, is a worldwide trend. Students still find themselves in difficulty, as their study time must also be allocated to other, more daunting, sub-specialty subjects, such as psychiatry, that are often grouped within this block.

The authors present multiple-choice questions covering all areas of ENT, grouped in the major divisions. This is an excellent means of preparation for medical undergraduate examinations, as gaps in core knowledge are quickly revealed. Furthermore, this text is a good guide for students who wish to identify those subject areas that require more focused study, especially when time is limited. This is a common problem among the undergraduates that I tutor. This book is for them.

Samir Soma MBChB(Pret) FCORL(SA)
Consultant Otorhinolaryngologist
Chris Hani Baragwanath Hospital
Soweto, Johannesburg
South Africa
Lecturer
Division of Otorhinolaryngology
Department of Neurosciences
Health Sciences Faculty
University of the Witwatersrand
March 2010

Preface

The subject of ear, nose and throat (ENT) surgery has traditionally been a difficult and specialised one for medical students, junior doctors and other healthcare professionals. Many textbooks on the topic are too detailed for undergraduate use, and many books written for medical students lack self-assessment questions. It was this problem faced by students which led the authors to write this book. This new, concise and easy-to-read self-assessment guide aims to elucidate this complex topic by means of easy-to-understand points that will help the reader to identify gaps in their understanding and then provide them with succinct explanations. It will also serve as a useful companion for clinics and teaching sessions.

The aim of this book is therefore to provide a comprehensive and detailed self-directed assessment of ENT for medical students, in the form of short succinct multiple-choice questions that cover a wide range of topics. The book is targeted at medical students of all years, will be of maximum benefit during preparation for end-of-unit/module/firm exams in ENT, and provides a solid basis for revision in ENT for the written finals. It will be of benefit for both standard undergraduate and graduate-entry medical curricula. It was written with a view to covering the learning objectives of most of the UK medical school curricula, and will be of great benefit to any medical student who is unsure of the standard expected for finals, or who wishes to identify gaps in their knowledge during revision.

The questions cover all levels of knowledge, from beginners to experts. The MCQs in this book will examine a detailed understanding of the topic and ensure confidence and competence when approaching examinations.

Gurdeep Singh Mannu
Tunde Odutoye
March 2010

About the authors

Gurdeep Singh Mannu graduated with a BSc (Hons) in anatomy and human sciences from King's College London. He obtained his MBBS from St George's, University of London, where he was actively involved in the teaching of medical students. He has a keen interest in the training of medical undergraduates, and is currently working as a foundation doctor at Norfolk and Norwich Hospital.

Tunde Odutoye is currently a consultant otolaryngologist and head and neck surgeon at St George's Hospital, University of London. He has a keen interest in clinical research and audit, especially with regard to quality of life, and treatment outcome issues for head and neck cancer patients. He is actively involved in ENT academia, and has a wealth of experience in the teaching of medical students.

How to use this book

The study of ENT can initially prove quite difficult for the student. The breadth of knowledge required for this specialised area can appear daunting. However, comfort can be derived from the fact that learning the basic principles of anatomy and physiology for the ear, nose and throat goes a long way towards overcoming much of the difficulty.

This book can be used either as a primary study companion or as a revision resource. Attempting the questions and working through them can be of benefit, as learning from mistakes by reading the explanation of the answer to each question helps one to remember the salient points. However, the best advice that can be given to readers would be to consult any of the many standard ENT undergraduate textbooks in order to gain a basic knowledge of the subject. This book can then be used to test one's basic understanding and to identify gaps in one's knowledge. This will be a more effective exercise, and the explanations of the answers to the questions can help to reinforce background knowledge.

During preparation for exams, this book can be used as a practice or 'mock' paper. It can be attempted under timed conditions and marked afterwards. This will help the reader to get a better idea of the time constraints of the approaching examination, as well as the style of examination question that they may encounter. The primary focus of this book is to provide a self-assessment guide for the student. As such it is not intended to replace a standard textbook, but rather to complement the student's personal study.

Finally, there is an old German proverb which states that 'a teacher is better than two books.' To fully appreciate and understand the subject, it is necessary to see and speak to the patients who are suffering from the conditions described in this book. Any number of books cannot replace attendance at outpatient clinics, surgical theatre sessions and inpatient ward rounds. Students will find that a small investment of time in any of these learning opportunities will pay rich dividends when they are trying to remember the details of a condition in the examination hall!

Good luck!

We would like to thank all of our friends and family who have supported and inspired this book.

The ear

Questions

1. With regard to Ménière's disease, the following statements are true:
   a It typically presents between the ages of 30 and 50 years.
   b It is characterised by the triad of hyperacusis, vertigo and tinnitus.
   c Treatment involves lifestyle changes such as a low-salt diet and the medical addition of a thiazide diuretic.
   d Audiometry will show a conductive hearing loss.
   e It can cause drop attacks.

2. Causes of dizziness include the following:
   a Ménière's disease.
   b Acute otitis media.
   c Cardiac arrhythmia.
   d Long-standing poorly controlled diabetes.
   e Migraine.

3. With regard to labyrinthitis, the following statements are true:
   a It can be a complication of upper respiratory tract infections.
   b It may cause hearing loss.
   c There is nystagmus towards the affected ear.
   d Vestibular suppressants are used in treatment.
   e It may be caused by viruses or bacteria.

4. With regard to vestibular neuronitis, the following statements are true:
   a Like labyrinthitis, vestibular neuronitis follows an upper respiratory tract infection.
   b It affects women more often than men.
   c If left untreated, it may go on to cause permanent deafness.
   d On examination, nystagmus may be elicited towards the affected ear.
   e Antiviral drugs are the mainstay of treatment.

5. With regard to Ramsay Hunt syndrome, the following statements are true:
    a It may present with facial palsy, hearing loss and vertigo.
    b It can be differentiated from Bell's palsy by the presence of cutaneous vesicles in the ear canal.
    c It is caused by adenovirus.
    d It may be treated with acyclovir and prednisolone.
    e It has an excellent prognosis, and 99% of patients regain premorbid facial nerve function.

6. With regard to benign paroxysmal positional vertigo (BPPV), the following statements are true:
    a It may present with severe vertigo when facing a certain direction.
    b Symptoms may be elicited by the Dix–Hallpike manoeuvre.
    c It is caused by the presence of an otolith moving within the semicircular canals.
    d It may be treated by the Epley manoeuvre.
    e BPPV originating from the horizontal and posterior semicircular canals can be differentiated by inspection of the respective type of nystagmus.

7. With regard to acoustic neuroma, the following statements are true:
    a It is a vestibular nerve Schwann cell neoplasm.
    b It is a fast-growing and deadly cancer if missed.
    c It may present with hearing loss and vertigo.
    d It is usually treated by chemotherapy.
    e It has an incidence of less than 1 in 100 000.

8. The following drugs are known to be ototoxic:
    a Gentamicin.
    b Some chemotherapy drugs.
    c Cimetidine.
    d Aspirin.
    e Quinine.

9. The causes of conductive hearing loss include the following:
    a Cholesteatoma.
    b Acoustic neuroma.
    c Presbycusis.
    d Otosclerosis.
    e Benign paroxysmal positional vertigo (BPPV).

10. Treatments for excess cerumen (ear wax) include the following:
    a Regular use of a cotton bud to ensure deep cleaning.
    b Irrigation.
    c The use of cerumenolytic agents.
    d Direct visual removal of cerumen using an otomicroscope.
    e Blind removal in primary care.

11. An HIV-positive patient presents with deep boring ear pain and a red inflamed ear canal and pinna. The following statements are true:
    a This is most likely to be a case of necrotising otitis externa.
    b The most likely cause is the pathogen *Pseudomonas aeruginosa*.
    c This should be treated conservatively with rest and topical hygiene.
    d Mortality of untreated cases may be one in every five patients.
    e This condition may cause a facial nerve palsy.

12. With regard to cochlear implants, the following statements are true:
    a The human ear is capable of detecting sound within the frequency range 20–20000 Hz.
    b The implants work by amplifying sound.
    c Cochlear implants are used in patients who are suffering from mild to moderate sensorineural hearing loss.
    d Patients who receive cochlear implants are at a higher risk of meningitis.
    e The majority of profound deafness is congenital in nature.

13. With regard to presbycusis, the following statements are true:
    a It has a higher prevalence in people of Afro-Caribbean origin.
    b It presents as unilateral sensorineural hearing loss, starting with high-frequency sound.
    c It may be treated with a hearing aid.
    d A patient with this condition will present with a reduced ability to differentiate consonants rather than vowels.
    e The aetiology of this condition is thought to be due to the degeneration of the tiny hair cells in the cochlea.

14. Causes of tinnitus include the following:
    a Furosemide.
    b Exposure to loud noise.
    c Benign paroxysmal positional vertigo.
    d Ménière's disease.
    e Multiple sclerosis.

15. With regard to autoimmune hearing loss, the following statements are true:
    a It presents as a gradual bilateral sensorineural hearing loss.
    b The condition improves with the use of steroids.
    c It may present with fluctuating sensorineural hearing loss, tinnitus and vertigo.
    d It is more common in men.
    e Immunosuppressants may be helpful.

16. With regard to mastoiditis, the following statements are true:
    a It can develop as a complication of otitis media.
    b If left untreated, mastoiditis can result in meningitis and facial nerve palsy.
    c Antibiotics are the mainstay of treatment.
    d Myringotomy should be avoided, due to the risk of further infection.
    e Mastoiditis is an indication for mastoidectomy.

17. With regard to cholesteatoma, the following statements are true:
    a It can be caused by squamous epithelium that is abnormally confined in the temporal or mastoid bone.
    b Replication of squamous epithelium causes destruction of its containing bone.
    c It may result in meningitis and brain abscess.
    d It usually presents with a painful discharge from the ear along with hearing loss.
    e Treatment is with systemic antibiotics.

18. With regard to otosclerosis, the following statements are true:
    a It has no ethnic predominance.
    b It results in a sensorineural hearing loss.
    c It may be inherited genetically.
    d Myringotomy may provide symptomatic relief.
    e It affects men more often than women.

19. With regard to perilymphatic fistula, the following statements are true:
    a It is an abnormal connection between the inner ear and the outer ear.
    b It chiefly presents with discharge from the ear.
    c Audiometry demonstrates a conductive hearing loss.
    d Surgical intervention is the only definitive treatment.
    e Patients may complain of an altered sense of taste following surgical intervention for this condition.

20. With regard to tympanic perforation, the following statements are true:
    a It most commonly occurs as a result of surgery.
    b It must not be treated conservatively.
    c It usually presents with ear discharge.
    d Hearing loss may be worsened as a complication of surgical intervention for tympanic perforation.
    e It is an indication for the use of high-dose topical gentamicin.

21. With regard to the ear, the following statements are true:
    a The ear can be divided into three compartments.
    b The tympanic membrane separates the outer ear from the middle ear.
    c The Eustachian tube opens into the middle ear.
    d The three sound-conducting ear bones or ossicles are found in the inner ear.
    e The cochlea is found in the middle ear.

22. With regard to accessory auricles, the following statements are true:
    a They often contain cartilage.
    b They are found along the intersection between the tragus and the angle of the mouth.
    c There may be more than one present.
    d They cause hearing loss.
    e They become cancerous if left untreated.

23. With regard to pre-auricular sinuses, the following statements are true:
    a They have an incidence of about 1%.
    b If left untreated, the associated mortality is about 30%.
    c They are more common in people of Asian and African origin.
    d They are commonly infected by *Staphylococcus* bacteria.
    e After surgical intervention, 20% of all cases re-occur.

24. With regard to pinna haematoma, the following statements are true:
  a It is usually caused by trauma which results in bleeding into the subperichondrial layer.
  b Ideally it should be left to resolve spontaneously.
  c It can result in the remodelling of the pinna to form a cauliflower ear.
  d The area affected by the haematoma should not be compressed or placed under pressure if the haematoma is evacuated.
  e Patients who present 8 days after the onset of a pinna haematoma are not amenable to aspiration treatment.

25. With regard to the external acoustic meatus of the outer ear, the following statements are true:
  a The external auditory canal is lined by columnar epithelium.
  b It is innervated by the trigeminal nerve.
  c The epithelial cells located here migrate towards the tympanic membrane.
  d The eardrum is located in an oblique position.
  e The ear canal is lined by ceruminous glands throughout its course.

26. With regard to otitis externa, the following statements are true:
  a Otitis externa is defined as inflammation of the outer ear.
  b Movement of the pinna is not usually painful.
  c First-line treatment should be systemic antibiotics.
  d Diabetes can give rise to malignant otitis externa.
  e The ear should be washed thoroughly daily, both morning and evening.

27. With regard to otitis media, the following statements are true:
  a Otitis media is defined as inflammation of the inner ear.
  b This condition is clinically diagnosed by the onset of pain on moving the pinna.
  c It is important to inspect behind the ear at the mastoid for redness and tenderness.
  d Treatment of otitis media should involve topical antibiotics.
  e The patient may complain of tinnitus and hearing loss.

28. With regard to grommets, the following statements are true:
    a A grommet is a small plastic tube that is inserted into the tympanic membrane.
    b Once a grommet is in place, swimming must be strictly avoided.
    c Grommets must be surgically removed or replaced after 5 to 6 months.
    d Permanent grommets will stay in place for the rest of the patient's life.
    e When grommets fall out, they usually leave behind a residual tympanic membrane perforation.

29. With regard to commonly used nomenclature in audiology, which of the following descriptions are true?
    a Otalgia refers to ear pain.
    b Otorrhoea refers to reddening of the ear.
    c Pure tone audiograms are a form of audiometry.
    d Tinnitus is the term used to describe discharge from the ear.
    e Aural drops consist of medicine that is delivered via drops into the mouth.

30. With regard to the cochlea, which of the following statements are true?
    a It is completely embedded in the temporal bone.
    b It is divided into three canals along its length by membranes.
    c The scala media is filled with perilymph fluid.
    d The scala vestibuli and scala tympani meet at the apical end of the cochlea, called the helicotrema.
    e The stapes is set in the round window, which conducts sound waves along the scala vestibuli.

31. With regard to the organ of Corti, which of the following statements are true?
    a It consists of Corti cells/hair cells, supporting cells, nerve terminals and the tectorial membrane.
    b It lies on Reissner's membrane within the cochlear ducts.
    c In humans there are about 3500 inner hair cells in each ear.
    d The outer hair cells provide most of the auditory input to the brain via cranial nerve VIII.
    e The inner hair cells receive major efferent input from the superior olivary complex.

32. Factors that will reduce effective communication with a deaf patient include the following:
    a   Covering the lips with the fingers or a hand while speaking.
    b   Poor lighting.
    c   Not facing the patient while speaking.
    d   Making good eye contact.
    e   Using accessory means of communication, such as writing, drawing or using sign language.

33. The following are cranial nerves that run within the middle ear:
    a   A branch of the facial nerve.
    b   A branch of the olfactory nerve.
    c   A branch of the glossopharyngeal nerve.
    d   A branch of the optic nerve.
    e   A branch of the trochlear nerve.

34. The following are bones involved in the conduction of sound in the middle ear:
    a   Stapes.
    b   Hamate.
    c   Malleus.
    d   Capitate.
    e   Incus.

35. When interpreting the results of Rinne and Weber tests, the following inferences are true:
  a If air conduction (AC) is greater than bone conduction (BC) bilaterally, and Weber testing is central, there may be normal hearing.
  b There is normal hearing in the right ear. However, in the left ear bone conduction is greater than air conduction, with Weber testing localising to the left. This may be due to conductive hearing loss in the left ear.
  c Air conduction is greater than bone conduction bilaterally. However, if Weber testing localises to the right, there may be right sensorineural hearing loss.
  d Bone conduction is greater than air conduction in the left ear, whereas air conduction is greater than bone conduction in the right ear. Weber testing localises to the right ear. The right ear was unmasked during the test. This suggests conductive hearing loss in the left ear.
  e Bone conduction is greater than air conduction bilaterally. Weber testing is central. This may suggest bilateral conductive hearing loss.

36. With regard to squamous-cell carcinoma of the pinna, the following statements are true:
  a The pinna is a common site for this cancer.
  b Treatment involves a wide local excision.
  c It tends to have a pearly white centre.
  d It can be treated with antibiotics.
  e It should not be treated, as the cancer will die naturally due to lack of blood supply.

37. The following are names of surgical ear operations:
  a Myringotomy.
  b Myomectomy.
  c Stapedectomy.
  d Appendicectomy.
  e Mastoidectomy.

38. The following may be non-otological (non-ear-related) causes of otalgia (ear pain):
a Cervical spondylosis.
b Osteoarthritis of the right knee.
c Sinusitis.
d Tonsillitis.
e Epistaxis.

39. When preparing a patient for ear surgery, the following investigations are routinely performed:
a FBC.
b LFT.
c Barium swallow.
d Technetium scan.
e U&Es.

40. With regard to a foreign body within the ear canal, which of the following statements are true?
a If it has not been removed on the first attempt, multiple attempts should be made in order to reduce the likelihood that removal under general anaesthetic will be necessary.
b Plastic foreign bodies in the ear are more serious than batteries.
c Suction can be used to extract the object.
d The object should be pushed as far as possible into the ear canal to allow the body to expel it naturally.
e Irrigation can be used to extract the object.

41. With regard to pinnaplasty, the following statements are true:
a It is an operation to correct prominent ears.
b Ideally, pinnaplasty should be performed in neonates.
c The operation lasts 6 to 7 hours and requires an intensive hospital stay of 7 days post-surgery.
d Patients should wear a head bandage for 7 days after surgery.
e A possible complication is haematoma formation.

42. The following are possible complications of a cholesteatoma:
a Dysphagia.
b Deafness.
c Epistaxis.
d Mastoiditis.
e Facial nerve palsy.

43. With regard to labyrinthitis, the following statements are true:
   a It is commonly caused by bacteria.
   b It presents with vertigo.
   c Symptoms are exacerbated by movement.
   d The eyes may demonstrate nystagmus.
   e It is diagnosed by recording an audiogram.

44. With regard to exostoses, which of the following statements are true?
   a They are more common in swimmers.
   b They are a direct cause of vertigo.
   c They can cause the impaction of ear wax.
   d They can be surgically removed.
   e They may present with conductive hearing loss.

45. Which of the following statements about hearing aids are true?
   a They amplify sound to help those with hearing impairment.
   b They can be divided into analogue and digital types.
   c They are of great benefit to patients suffering from presbycusis.
   d They can have life-changing effects on a person's quality of life.
   e They are not available on the National Health Service.

46. Which of the following are components of a standard hearing aid?
   a A processor.
   b A recording/storage hard drive.
   c A microphone.
   d A printer.
   e A transmitter.

47. With regard to chronic suppurative otitis media, which of the following statements are true?
   a There may be discharge from the affected ear (otorrhoea).
   b It has a poor prognosis.
   c It may result in cholesteatoma formation.
   d There may be hearing loss in the affected ear.
   e There may be a history of recurrent otitis media.

48. With regard to bullous myringitis, which of the following statements are true?
a It is a form of acute otitis media.
b It may be caused by viral or bacterial infection.
c It is characterised by vesicles on the tympanic membrane.
d It is commonly painless.
e It is diagnosed by CT scan.

49. Which of the following patients would not benefit from the use of an analogue 'over-the-ear' hearing aid?
a A 78-year-old woman with severe rheumatoid arthritis in her hands.
b A 62-year-old woman who has been pressured or coerced into requesting a hearing aid by her family.
c A 52-year-old woman with mild to moderate presbycusis.
d A 6-year-old boy with negligible cochlear function.
e A 22-year-old man with normal hearing who complains of tinnitus after leaving a club where loud music is playing.

50. A 22-year-old woman comes to see you with bilateral progressive hearing loss. She claims that this started in her teens, and she now complains of tinnitus. On auroscope examination you note a pink but otherwise normal tympanic membrane. Which of the following are true regarding this condition?
a This patient is suffering from acute otitis media.
b Her condition may be genetically inherited.
c This patient may be suffering from otosclerosis.
d She may benefit from a hearing aid.
e She may benefit from surgery.

51. Which of the following may be causes of acute otitis externa?
a Carbon dioxide.
b Asbestos.
c Viral herpes infection.
d Fungal infection.
e Bacterial infection.

52. Which of the following may result in sensorineural hearing loss?
a Meningitis.
b Chemotherapy.
c Cholesteatoma.
d Neonatal hypoxia.
e Acute otitis media.

53. Which of the following statements are true with regard to localised basal-cell carcinoma of the ear?
  a It has a pearly white appearance.
  b It is treated with chemotherapy in the first instance.
  c It is more likely to metastasise than other skin cancers.
  d It is usually bloody with a granular appearance.
  e It requires wide local excision.

54. Which of the following are functions of the Eustachian tube?
  a It allows coughing.
  b It drains cerumen from the outer ear.
  c It allows the drainage of secretions from the middle ear.
  d It allows sneezing.
  e It is responsible for pressure regulation in the middle ear.

55. A 21-year-old man attends your ENT clinic with recurrent otitis media and a red painful swelling behind the ear. The consultant informs you that the patient has mastoiditis. Which of the following are possible complications of this condition?
  a Lung cancer.
  b Intracranial abscess.
  c Irritable bowel syndrome.
  d Osteitis.
  e Laryngeal stenosis.

56. Which of the following may be involved in the management of mastoiditis following otitis media?
  a No treatment other than fluids and rest.
  b Intravenous antibiotics.
  c Mastoidectomy.
  d Defibrillation.
  e A nasal tampon.

57. Which of the following are causes of progressive hearing loss?
  a Parotitis.
  b Long-term use of ototoxic medication.
  c Genetic causes.
  d Sudden head trauma.
  e Long-term exposure to loud noise.

58. Which of the following difficulties may face a child with pre-lingual deafness?
    a Delayed social development.
    b Swallowing difficulties.
    c Social isolation.
    d Delayed motor development.
    e Irritability, aggression or depression.

59. When communicating with a patient with sensorineural hearing loss, which of the following should be considered?
    a You should shout as loudly as possible next to their ear.
    b You should speak as slowly as possible to help the patient to lip-read.
    c You should stand opposite the patient and maintain good eye contact.
    d You could use a sign language interpreter.
    e You should draw diagrams to explain your point.

60. Your clinic is running very late, and the next patient is an adult with sudden-onset acquired sensorineural hearing loss. With regard to communication with this patient, which of the following statements are true?
    a Written information is useful to help to educate the patient.
    b It is best to speak to the relative and ask them to explain the consultation to the patient when they get home.
    c Sign language must be used.
    d You should shout as loudly as possible next to their ear.
    e This patient should not be allocated any additional time due to the communication difficulties involved, and should be hurried as other patients are waiting.

61. Which of the following are features indicative of a poor prognosis in a patient with sudden hearing loss?
    a Ear pain following a recent cold.
    b Bilateral hearing loss.
    c Vertigo.
    d Age less than 15 years.
    e Severe hearing loss.

62. Syringing of the ear is used to remove wax. Which of the following statements are true regarding this technique?
    a Before syringing, the wax should be softened using cerumenolytics.
    b Water should be at –1°C in order to break up the wax effectively.
    c The syringe should be aimed downwards and forwards in the ear canal.
    d Water should be at 37–38°C to remove the wax effectively.
    e The syringe should be aimed upwards and backwards in the ear canal.

63. A 22-year-old woman presents to you with earache. On examination you elicit pain by pressing on the tragus, and on auroscope examination you can see that the ear canal is very inflamed. After you have explained the diagnosis of otitis externa to the patient, she asks what she can do to avoid this happening again in the future. Which of the following answers to her question are true?
    a Try to protect the ear when bathing or showering.
    b Avoid swimming in dirty water.
    c Ensure that you rigorously wash out the affected ear in the shower.
    d Drink plenty of cranberry juice.
    e Do not use cotton buds to clean your ear.

64. In the management of otitis externa, which of the following measures may be used?
    a Washing out the affected ear daily with soapy water.
    b Analgesia.
    c Avoiding listening to loud music.
    d Antibiotics.
    e Preventive measures to keep the ear canal clean.

65. Which of the following pathogens may directly cause otitis externa?
    a *Candida albicans.*
    b *Pseudomonas aeruginosa.*
    c Rhinovirus.
    d *Staphylococcus aureus.*
    e *Aspergillus* species.

66. Which of the following groups of patients are more susceptible to malignant otitis externa?
    a Those with HIV infection.
    b Patients with severe asthma who are taking excessive amounts of steroids.
    c Those with diabetes.
    d Patients undergoing chemotherapy.
    e The elderly.

67. Which of the following are symptoms of malignant otitis externa?
    a Itchy ear.
    b Otorrhoea.
    c Coughing.
    d Hearing loss.
    e Painful ear.

68. A 62-year-old man comes to see you complaining of frequent bouts of dizziness and fainting when looking up and over his shoulder. He occasionally experiences diplopia and headaches. There is no hearing loss and no nystagmus elicited by the Dix–Hallpike manoeuvre. When you ask him to look up, he drops to the floor unconscious. Which of the following conditions is this patient suffering from?
    a Ménière's disease.
    b Labyrinthitis.
    c Benign paroxysmal positional vertigo.
    d Perilymphatic fistula.
    e Vertebrobasilar insufficiency.

69. A mother brings her 6-year-old boy to see you. She claims that he has been holding his ear often over the past couple of days, and that he is not himself today. She goes on to explain that he has been irritable and has developed a rash, which she believes to be an allergy to the Calpol that she has been giving him. You notice that the child has a non-blanching rash and is photophobic. He has a high-pitched cry with neck stiffness. Which of the following statements are true?
    a The child must be given metronidazole immediately.
    b This is a complication of his acute otitis media.
    c The mother should be reassured that there is nothing to worry about and sent home.
    d The child must be given ceftriaxone immediately.
    e The condition is untreatable, and palliative care should be started.

70. Which of the following congenital infections can result in deafness?
a *Staphylococcus*.
b Syphilis.
c Rubella.
d Candida.
e Cytomegalovirus.

71. Which of the following are true of acute bacterial parotitis?
a There is a swelling under the chin.
b It commonly results in acute otitis externa.
c There is a swelling in the region of the cheek.
d It is alleviated by nasal decongestants.
e Pain is made worse by chewing.

72. Which of the following are true regarding chronic suppurative otitis media?
a It is a form of chronic otitis media.
b Patients have otorrhoea.
c Patients have sensorineural hearing loss.
d Patients always have a tympanic membrane perforation.
e Symptoms must last for more than 2 weeks for this diagnosis to be made.

73. Which of the following statements about the nomenclature used to describe chronic suppurative otitis media (CSOM) are true?
a CSOM with cholesteatoma is described as active.
b CSOM with cholesteatoma and infection is described as radioactive.
c CSOM with cholesteatoma and infection is described as unsafe.
d CSOM with cholesteatoma is described as safe.
e CSOM with no infection is described as safe.

74. Regarding serous otitis media, which of the following statements are true?
a It may present with hearing loss.
b It may result from Eustachian tube blockage.
c In children, it may get better with age.
d There is always tympanic membrane perforation.
e Antihistamines may be helpful.

75. Which of the following may be causes of Eustachian tube blockage?
    a   An anatomically different Eustachian tube in children to that in adults.
    b   Adenoid hypertrophy.
    c   An enlarged tongue.
    d   Infection.
    e   Acute otitis externa.

76. Regarding cholesteatoma, which of the following statements are true?
    a   It is a cancer.
    b   It should be left untreated.
    c   It consists of columnar epithelium.
    d   It may metastasise to distant sites.
    e   It is mainly treated medically.

77. A patient has recently been diagnosed with cholesteatoma, but is reluctant to have surgical treatment. He wishes to speak to you regarding the complications of this condition if it remains untreated. The following are complications of untreated cholesteatoma:
    a   Dizziness.
    b   Deafness.
    c   Hyperthyroidism.
    d   Facial paralysis.
    e   Meningitis.

78. The following are indications for the insertion of a grommet:
    a   Laryngeal cancer.
    b   Glue ear.
    c   Parotitis.
    d   Adenoid hypertrophy.
    e   Recurrent severe otitis media.

79. Regarding the hair cells of the ear, which of the following statements are true?
    a   They are mechanoreceptors.
    b   They consist of several large kinocilia and several thousand stereocilia.
    c   The tip of the stereocilium is bathed in perilymph.
    d   The body of the hair cell is bathed in endolymph.
    e   Mechanical deformation against the kinocilium opens potassium channels in the stereocilia.

80. Which of the following middle ear structures are derived from the first pharyngeal arch?
    a The incus bone.
    b The stapes bone.
    c The malleus bone.
    d The thyroid cartilage.
    e The thymus.

81. Which of the following medical terms is coupled with its correct description?
    a Microtia refers to large ears.
    b Anotia refers to a third ear.
    c Synotia is the term used to describe ears that are too close to the midline anteriorly.
    d Melotia refers to an ear arising from the cheek.
    e Macrotia is the term used to describe a large tongue.

82. Which of the following statements about vertigo are true?
    a It is a sensation of motion in any direction when the body is stationary.
    b It is a sensation of spinning only.
    c It is one of a triad of symptoms of Ménière's disease, the others being headache and vomiting.
    d It may be relieved in certain situations by the Epley manoeuvre.
    e It can occur due to mismatched sensory inputs from the eyes, ears, and muscle and joint proprioceptors.

83. The following statements about ear wax are true:
    a The ear should be cleaned out and wax removed on a regular basis.
    b Cotton buds are a good tool for removing wax.
    c Ear wax is produced by glands in the skin only in the outer half of the ear canal.
    d The consistency varies among different races and ethnic groups.
    e It can cause deafness if impacted in the ear canal.

The ear

Answers

1. a **True.** It commonly presents in middle age.

   b **False.** Ménière's disease is characterised by the triad of vertigo, tinnitus and sensorineural hearing loss. Hyperacuism (heightened hearing) is not a feature of this condition. In Ménière's disease there are intermittent attacks of these three symptoms, lasting for up to a couple of hours, before resolving gradually over a couple of days.

   c **True.** Treatment initially involves lifestyle changes, including a low-salt diet, a reduction in caffeine intake, and smoking cessation. Medical treatment includes the addition of a thiazide diuretic. Reduction in salt intake and diuretic use is based on the theory that an abnormal electrolyte balance in the vestibular labyrinth is a cause of the disease. Other theories suggest the presence of excess endolymph in the labyrinth through a different method.

   Surgical treatment involves techniques such as vestibular nerve section. Acute attacks can be treated with vestibular suppressants. However, the long-term final and definitive treatment is the use of sensorineural toxic aminoglycosides. These drugs will cure the vertigo and tinnitus, but will result in irreversible sensorineural hearing loss.

   d **False.** Audiometry will demonstrate sensorineural hearing loss in Ménière's disease, not a conductive hearing loss.

   e **True.** Patients with late-stage disease may suddenly lose all tone and collapse fully conscious on to the ground during abrupt attacks.

2. When taking a history of dizziness, care must be taken to specifically differentiate vertigo from light-headedness. Vertigo is the abnormal feeling of movement, or a hallucination of movement, which thus distinguishes it from faintness or lightheadedness. It

can be in any direction, but is usually described as a spinning or rotatory motion. Once the complaint has been clarified, specific features in the history can help to elucidate the diagnosis further. These include the presence or absence of associated features (e.g. palpitations, tinnitus, hearing loss, ear pain or headache) in addition to the particular details of the episode (e.g. the timing and possible cause of dizziness). Finally, enquiry into the patient's general health is often productive, especially if there has been a recent infection favouring the diagnosis of labyrinthitis, or a background of osteoarthritis (possibly resulting in vertebrobasilar insufficiency) or heart disease (resulting in a cardiac arrhythmia).

Dizziness or vertigo may be associated with or exacerbated by a range of activities, from standing up quickly (in postural hypotension) to facing a certain direction (in benign paroxysmal positional vertigo). There may be clues in the medication history suggesting long-standing conditions such as diabetes and hypertension. Neurological conditions must be probed for, and there must be general screening for metabolic and neoplasmic causes (e.g. acoustic neuroma, paraneoplastic syndrome, Addison's disease and hypothyroidism). The answers to the above questions are as follows:

a **True.**
b **True.**
c **True.**
d **True.**
e **True.**

3. a **True.** Labyrinthitis describes inflammation of the labyrinth. It follows an upper respiratory tract infection in around 50% of cases.
   b **True.** Patients who present with labyrinthitis characteristically complain of hearing loss and vertigo.
   c **False.** On examination you may find that the patient has nystagmus towards the unaffected ear, not the affected ear.
   d **True.** Vestibular suppressant and anti-emetic medication can be used for symptomatic relief. With rest and conservative measures, labyrinthitis usually resolves spontaneously over a period of 1 or 2 weeks. It may take up to 6 months to resolve in older people, and can sometimes lead to recurring attacks. For bacterial causes, antibiotics based on sensitivities may be used. For viral causes, a short dose of steroids may be beneficial.

e **True.** There are a large number of pathogens that may cause labyrinthitis. Viral causes include respiratory syncytial virus, influenza virus and herpes virus. Bacterial causes include *Haemophilus influenzae*, and *Staphylococcus* and *Streptococcus* species.

4. a **False.** Vestibular neuronitis and labyrinthitis are commonly confused. This confusion is perpetuated when the two terms are used synonymously in books. Labyrinthitis follows an upper respiratory tract infection in over 50% of cases, as discussed previously. However, the cause of vestibular neuronitis is still largely unknown. The symptoms result from inflammation of the vestibular nerve. The latter is responsible for balance, so disruption of its function causes symptoms of nausea, vomiting and vertigo.

    b **False.** Vestibular neuronitis affects men and women equally. There is no gender predominance.

    c **False.** Vestibular neuronitis is a self-limiting, short-term illness that usually lasts for a few weeks. As mentioned above, the main symptoms are nausea, vomiting and vertigo. Since it affects only the vestibular nerve, it has no effect on hearing (which is innervated by the cochlear nerve). In rare cases, nausea and vertigo may occasionally occur some time after the initial illness.

    d **False.** As in labyrinthitis, patients suffering from vestibular neuronitis have nystagmus towards the unaffected ear, not towards the affected ear.

    e **False.** As there is little evidence that viral infection is the cause of vestibular neuronitis, antiviral medication is not the mainstay of treatment. High-dose steroids that are then gradually reduced over a period of 3 weeks have been shown to be beneficial in preventing the long-term sequelae of the disease.

5. a **True.** Ramsay Hunt syndrome is a collection of several symptoms. It usually presents with one-sided facial weakness with ipsilateral hearing loss and ear pain radiating outwards. Erythematous vesicles seen in the ear canal further narrow down the differential diagnosis. Patients may also complain of vertigo, and of tinnitus and pain when opening the mouth.

    b **True.** It is important to look in the ear canal of all patients who present with Bell's palsy. Around 20% of those patients who are diagnosed with Bell's palsy are actually suffering from Ramsay Hunt syndrome, which could easily have been detected with a simple auroscope examination.

c **False.** It is caused by herpes simplex virus type 3, not by adenovirus.

d **True.** Ramsay Hunt syndrome may be treated with a course of an antiviral medication and a corticosteroid. However, recent studies have shown that prednisolone alone has a superior prognosis at 6 months compared with that of an antiviral drug. Vestibular suppressants are helpful for symptomatic release in severe vertigo, nausea and vomiting.

e **False.** Despite treatment, less than 50% of patients will regain total premorbid facial nerve function. Care must be taken to teach patients about the condition, with particular emphasis on measures to protect the cornea from irritation and damage (since the syndrome means that the patient will be unable to completely close the ipsilateral eyelid).

6. a **True.** It can present with sudden severe vertigo when turning over in bed, or turning to face a particular direction.

b **True.** This is a manoeuvre performed when BPPV is suspected. The patient sits on the examination bed as the examiner gently supports the patient, laying them on their back with their head to one side and hanging over the end of the bed. The examiner then inspects for nystagmus. In a positive test the patient will complain of vertigo and exhibit nystagmus during this manoeuvre.

c **True.** This is the most widely accepted theory with regard to the aetiology of BPPV. It describes small calcium carbonate particles that are free-floating in the semicircular canal. Any sudden movement will cause them to affect the natural endolymph flow and result in stimulation of the tiny hairs that are afferent to the vestibular nerve. This explains the sudden onset of vertigo experienced by the patient when turning to face a particular direction.

d **True.** This is a specific manoeuvre that involves asking the patient to move their head and body to specific positions. The Epley manoeuvre is performed to help to move the calcium carbonate deposits from the canals. This manoeuvre is contraindicated in patients with arthritic neck disease and in those with neurological problems, such as a past history of stroke.

e **True.** BPPV has a rotatory horizontal nystagmus in particular positions of the head shortly after head movement. The type of nystagmus provides further diagnostic information about the position of the calcium carbonate deposit.

7. a **True.**
   b **False.** It is a benign neoplasm that can be deadly if left untreated. However, it tends to grow relatively slowly.
   c **True.** Unilateral hearing loss is the classic presentation of acoustic neuroma. However, vertigo may also occur less commonly.
   d **False.** After MRI imaging, surgical excision or radiotherapy is the technique of choice for treatment of an acoustic neuroma. Chemotherapy does not have a role in the treatment of this disease.
   e **True.** However, recent research suggests that the true number of undetected acoustic neuromas may be 20 times this number!

8. a **True.** Ototoxic means 'toxic to the ear.' Aminoglycoside antibiotics are well known to be ototoxic, and for this reason are used in the treatment of severe Ménière's disease.
   b **True.** Some chemotherapy used in the treatment of cancer is well known to be ototoxic (e.g. cisplatin).
   c **False.** Cimetidine is an antihistamine and is not known to be ototoxic. The other common ototoxic drug of which it is important to be aware, and that is omitted from this list, is the diuretic furosemide.
   d **True.** Aspirin should not be used in children, due to the well-documented Reye's syndrome.
   e **True.** Quinines are ototoxic in high doses.

9. a **True.** Cholesteatoma is an abnormal benign growth of epithelial cells, and can cause conductive hearing loss.
   b **False.** Acoustic neuroma is a neoplasm of the Schwann cells surrounding the vestibular nerve. It results in a sensorineural hearing loss, not a conductive hearing loss.
   c **False.** Presbycusis is the natural degeneration of hearing with age, and is not a type of conductive hearing loss. It is by definition a type of sensorineural hearing loss.
   d **True.** Otosclerosis commonly occurs in young people, and is responsible for a progressive conductive hearing loss. It is caused by abnormal growth of the small ossicle bones in the middle ear, as a result of which they become immobile and cause a conductive hearing loss.
   e **False.** BPPV results in vertigo, but does not cause hearing loss.

10. a **False.** There is still widespread public misunderstanding about the use of cotton buds to attempt to maintain ear canal hygiene.

A cotton bud should not be used to clean the ear canal, as it only serves to push ear wax deeper into the canal, rather than actually removing it.

b **True.** Irrigation is a technique commonly used in primary care practice to treat cerumen-induced conductive hearing loss.

c **True.** Often simple olive oil is very effective in softening ear wax.

d **True.** It is important to clearly visualise the ear wax when removing it using an otomicroscope.

e **False.** Blind removal of cerumen should never be undertaken. Due to the lack of visual confirmation of the location of the curette, it can cause perforation and damage to the ear canal.

11. a **True.** Necrotising otitis externa should always be considered in immunocompromised individuals, such as patients suffering from AIDs, haematological malignancies or diabetes.

b **True.** *Pseudomonas aeruginosa* is the pathogen most commonly isolated in this condition.

c **False.** This is a serious condition, and it requires local debridement and intravenous antibiotics.

d **True.** Some studies suggest an even higher mortality rate! Always consider necrotising otitis externa in patients who present with symptoms of severe otitis externa but do not respond to topical treatment, and who have a past medical history of diabetes or an immunocompromised status.

e **True.** If this occurs, the patient is likely to have a poorer prognosis.

12. a **True.** Although the human ear is capable of detecting frequencies in the range 20–20 000 Hz, the upper extreme of this range deteriorates with age (due to a process known as presbycusis).

b **False.** Hearing aids work by amplifying sound. Cochlear implants work by directly stimulating the cochlear nerve, and thus bypassing the natural sound conduction process. The components of a cochlear implant consist of a microphone, processor and stimulator. The stimulator is placed in the cochlear apparatus and electrically stimulates the cochlear nerve. Modern cochlear implants have very advanced processors, which can even specifically focus on human speech.

c **False.** Cochlear implants are reserved for those patients who have moderate to profound sensorineural hearing loss.

d **True.** Patients who have cochlear implants are at higher risk of developing *Streptococcus pneumoniae* meningitis. For this reason these patients should receive the pneumococcal vaccine.

e **True.** The vast majority of profound sensorineural hearing loss occurs as a result of genetic mutations. It is important to detect hearing loss in babies and young children as soon as possible in order to prevent a detrimental effect on the child's development. Delayed developmental milestones are an important clue, and should prompt the physician to refer the child for hearing screening.

13. a **False.** There is no known ethnic predominance of this condition. The condition describes the natural loss of hearing with age. It is thus a disease of the elderly, with as many as one-third of patients aged 60 years experiencing some degree of hearing loss.

b **False.** Although presbycusis is defined by sensorineural hearing loss (starting with the higher-frequency range of sound), it is typically bilateral and does not present unilaterally. The main investigation in this condition is pure-tone audiometry.

c **True.** Hearing aids amplify sound, and so may prove to be of great benefit to patients with presbycusis.

d **True.** Normal speech can be divided into high-frequency and low-frequency sounds. The vowels make up the majority of low-frequency sounds, whereas consonants constitute high-frequency sound. Since presbycusis is initially manifested as a loss of high-frequency hearing, patients present with a reduced ability to differentiate consonants compared with vowels.

e **True.** Although this is thought to be the process, the actual underlying cause of this is still in dispute. Widely accepted causes include accumulative noise trauma, medical insults (e.g. ototoxic drugs), genetic causes and atherosclerotic risk factors (e.g. hypertension, smoking and high intake of saturated fats).

14. a **True.** Furosemide is an ototoxic drug that may cause tinnitus in high doses.

b **True.** Exposure to loud noise can result in a transient tinnitus (e.g. on entering a quiet area after leaving a room where loud music is playing). Continuous exposure to loud noise over a period of time can cumulatively result in noise-induced hearing loss.

c **False.** Benign paroxysmal positional vertigo is a vestibular problem. It presents with vertigo, nausea and vomiting following movement of the head in a particular direction. It does not affect the cochlear nerve and therefore does not cause tinnitus.

d **True.** Ménière's disease is characterised by the triad of sensorineural hearing loss, tinnitus and vertigo.

e **True.** Multiple sclerosis is a cause of tinnitus. In addition to the causes outlined in this question, tinnitus also has neurological causes (e.g. stroke) and cardiovascular causes (e.g. hypertension).

15. a **True.** Autoimmune hearing loss is a very interesting condition. It is diagnosed by subacute hearing loss. It is too slow to occur as a result of a sudden traumatic hearing loss, but its onset is too fast to be a result of natural degeneration with time (presbycusis).

b **True.** As is the case with most autoimmune conditions, steroids help in the management of this condition.

c **True.** The symptoms make it very difficult to distinguish from Ménière's disease. However, the fluctuating course of symptoms in autoimmune hearing loss distinguishes it from other differential diagnoses.

d **False.** As with most autoimmune conditions, autoimmune hearing loss is more common in women. This condition has associations with other autoimmune diseases that are also more common in women (e.g. systemic lupus erythematosus and rheumatoid arthritis).

e **True.** It is important to inform the patient about the benefits as well as the risks of immunosuppressive therapy. The patient must make an informed decision as to whether the treatment outcomes outweigh the risks. Examples of immunosuppressant therapies used in this condition include cyclophosphamide, methotrexate and azathioprine.

16. a **True.** Mastoiditis is a complication of middle ear infection. It can develop from chronic suppurative otitis media as well as acute otitis media.

b **True.** Meningitis is a serious complication, and testament to the reason why mastoiditis should be treated aggressively.

c **True.** Tissue or swab samples should be sent for microbial culture and antibiotic sensitivities. Ultimately, antibiotic therapy should be appropriate to the respective microbiological results.

d **False.** Myringotomy is a useful surgical intervention for relieving pain and patient discomfort in mastoiditis.

e **True.** Mastoiditis can lead to the formation of a subperiosteal abscess. If this is left untreated, it can result in the development of a brain abscess or meningitis. Consequently, mastoidectomy is an important therapeutic intervention. However, it is not without risks, and the patient should be informed about the possibility of facial deformity following surgery.

17. a **True.** This statement describes the aetiology of a congenital cholesteatoma. Acquired cholesteatomas can result from trauma, chronic infection or Eustachian tube dysfunction.

b **True.** This erosion of bone can form large avascular sinuses.

c **True.** Cholesteatomas can have life-threatening complications.

d **False.** Cholesteatomas do present with discharge from the ear and hearing loss. However, this is usually painless. The presence of pain would suggest an alternative diagnosis.

e **False.** The squamous epithelium is abnormally located within the bone. As a result, it has no blood supply and therefore systemic antibiotics will be unable to reach any infection located there. Treatment is by surgical removal of the cholesteatoma.

18. a **False.** Otosclerosis is more common in Caucasian people than in individuals of other ethnic origin. It is defined by the abnormal growth of bone at the ends of the small bones in the middle ear. This is what gives rise to the presentation of hearing loss.

b **False.** Otosclerosis presents with a slowly progressive conductive hearing loss, not a sensorineural hearing loss.

c **True.** Otosclerosis results from gene mutations that are inherited in an autosomal dominant pattern.

d **False.** Myringotomy has no role in the treatment of otosclerosis. It is used to relieve pressure in the middle ear caused by otitis media. The treatment of otosclerosis involves conservative measures such as the use of hearing aids, and surgical intervention with a stapedectomy, in which the abnormal stapes is replaced with a prosthesis, allowing more effective conduction of sound.

e **False.** Otosclerosis affects women twice as often as men.

19. a **False.** A perilymphatic fistula is an abnormal connection between the inner perilymphatic space and the mastoid or middle ear.

b **False.** A perilymphatic fistula presents with tinnitus, vertigo, hearing loss and a feeling of fullness within the ear. There is no visible discharge. Due to these symptoms it is very difficult to differentiate perilymphatic fistula from Ménière's disease on the basis of the clinical history alone.

c **False.** Sensorineural hearing loss is detected in patients who have a perilymphatic fistula, not conductive hearing loss.

d **True.** Surgical grafting at the site of the fistula is the only definitive treatment in patients with a perilymphatic fistula.

e **True.** This is as a result of damage to the chorda tympani during surgery, although most patients recover fully from this within a couple of months.

20. a **False.** Tympanic perforation most commonly occurs as a result of infection, notably acute otitis media or chronic suppurative otitis media. Trauma and surgery may also cause tympanic perforation, although less commonly.

 b **False.** Most small tympanic perforations will heal spontaneously without complications. In these patients a conservative approach to management is best. Hearing aids can be used to assist any subsequent hearing loss from the perforation, and medical treatment for the underlying cause of the perforation (e.g. systemic antibiotics for otitis media) is usually all that is necessary. Surgical treatment is reserved for those patients who have large perforations, and for those with prolonged, poorly healing perforations.

 c **True.** A common presentation of tympanic perforation is discharge from the ear, due to the inflammatory process that is occurring within the middle ear. If the patient has been suffering from pain due to otitis media, this is typically suddenly relieved when the tympanic membrane perforates. This perforation is characterised by a flow of discharge from the middle ear.

 d **True.** Unfortunately, one of the complications of surgical intervention for this condition is a subsequent exacerbation of hearing loss.

 e **False.** The ototoxicity of gentamicin is well documented, and it should be avoided in patients with tympanic perforation.

21. a **True.** The ear can be divided into the outer, middle and inner ear.

 b **True.**

 c **True.** The Eustachian tube or auditory canal connects the middle ear and the nasopharynx so as to equilibrate the pressure in the middle ear with the outside pressure.

 d **False.** The ossicles (i.e. malleus, incus and stapes) which connect the tympanic membrane to the cochlea are found in the middle ear.

 e **False.** The cochlea is located in the inner ear.

22. a **True.** Accessory auricles are embryological malformations that appear as small lobes of cartilaginous tissue.

b **True.** This is due to the embryological development of the ear.

c **True.**

d **False.** Accessory auricles do not cause hearing loss. Often they do not cause any problems other than cosmetic issues.

e **False.** Accessory auricles are benign and do not become cancerous if left untreated.

23. a **True.** The incidence varies according to ethnic origin. The incidence of preauricular sinus among Caucasians is less than 1%. The external ear develops from six embryological hillocks. Malformation of two of these hillocks (arising from the first and second branchial arches) during development is the cause of a preauricular sinus. Most patients present with an infection of the sinus, and the diagnosis should be suspected in patients with cellulitis of the region.

b **False.** A preauricular sinus is not a cause of mortality. They are usually treated for infection with antibiotics, and surgery is reserved for more symptomatic patients.

c **True.** The incidence is considerably higher in these populations compared with that among Caucasians.

d **True.** *Staphylococcus* bacteria are the cause of two-thirds of infected preauricular sinuses.

e **True.** Unfortunately, surgery for this condition has a high failure rate.

24. a **True.** A haematoma is common among individuals who engage in impact sports such as boxing and rugby. It results from bleeding into the subperichondrial layer.

b **False.** It requires rapid evacuation (within 7 days from the date of formation) to prevent fibrosis and the formation of a cauliflower ear.

c **True.** Fibrosis is the process by which a haematoma can cause reshaping of the ear into the visibly deformed cauliflower ear.

d **True.** It is by applying constant pressure after aspirating the haematoma that it can be prevented from reforming. It is important that the pressure applied is appropriate to the natural contours of the person's ear, otherwise the ear may still develop a deformity.

e **True.** Pinna haematoma can only be aspirated within a short time frame, up to 7 days from the onset of trauma. Patients who present with this condition after 7 days are not amenable to treatment by aspiration, as the process of fibrosis is not reversible after this stage.

25. a **False.** The external auditory canal is lined mainly by keratinising squamous epithelium. However, the tympanic membrane is lined by columnar epithelium on the inner aspect. It has a fibrous layer lateral to this and an outermost squamous epithelial layer.

  b **True.** The outer ear is partially innervated by the auriculo-temporal nerve, which is a branch of the trigeminal nerve (cranial nerve V). The ear canal is also supplied by branches from the vagus nerve. This nerve provides the afferent input to the ear–cough reflex, which explains why your patient may cough as you are examining their ear with your auroscope! The auricle is also supplied by the greater and lesser auricular nerves which arise from the C1–C3 cervical nerve roots.

  c **False.** The epithelial cells located in the outer ear actually migrate from the tympanic membrane outwards. This helps to move debris and wax naturally in an outward direction away from the tympanic membrane.

  d **True.** The tympanic membrane is positioned obliquely and attached by a fibrocartilaginous ring to the tympanic part of the temporal bone. It is the tympanic membrane that divides and separates the outer and middle ear.

  e **False.** The ear canal is only lined by ceruminous (wax) glands and hair in the outer cartilaginous third of its course. The inner two-thirds are lined by squamous cells in the bony meatus.

26. a **True.** Otitis externa is defined as inflammation of the outer ear, whereas otitis media refers to inflammation of the middle ear.

  b **False.** In otitis externa, movement of the pinna is characteristically painful. This helps to differentiate it from otitis media.

  c **False.** First-line treatment should involve suction of any debris from the external ear, followed by the administration of topical antibiotics in the form of ear drops.

  d **True.** Otitis externa in a diabetic patient is of particular concern, as these patients are at risk of a particularly severe form of the condition, known as malignant otitis externa. This is discussed in more detail in another question.

  e **False.** The patient should be instructed to ensure that the ear is kept dry, especially while washing or bathing. The ear itself should not be washed.

27. a **False.** Otitis media refers to inflammation of the middle ear.

  b **False.** In otitis media there is pain in the ear, but movement of the pinna does not affect this pain. This is in contrast to otitis externa, in which movement of the pinna characteristically causes pain. In otitis media there is a progressive increase in pain which is suddenly alleviated by discharge from the ear. This represents a perforation in the tympanic membrane that occurs as a result of the increased pressure in the middle ear caused by the inflammatory process.

c   **True.** A complication of otitis media is mastoiditis. This is a serious complication, and it will only be found if it is specifically searched for!

d   **False.** There must be a clear distinction between the treatment of otitis externa, which involves the use of topical antibiotics, and the treatment of otitis media, which involves the use of systemic antibiotics.

e   **True.** The classic presentation of otitis media involves a history of a recent upper respiratory tract infection or a cold, followed by unilateral hearing loss, tinnitus, and ear pain or possibly ear discharge. A full history should be taken with specific emphasis on whether this has happened before, whether the patient has any medical problems (e.g. diabetes) or any conditions that are associated with immunocompromised status, and which medication the patient is taking (e.g. steroids, immunosuppressant drugs). A full clinical examination should be performed to look for systemic signs of illness. An auroscope is an essential part of the examination. The tympanic membrane should be visualised, and may appear swollen, bulging, red and inflamed. A perforation may be visible.

28.   a   **True.** Grommets are normally used to relieve pressure in the middle ear in the case of glue ear, and to aerate the middle ear in the case of recurrent acute otitis media. The process of inserting a grommet is quite simple. A myringotomy is performed, which involves surgical perforation of the tympanic membrane, followed by suction of any infusion present in the middle ear before the grommet is inserted. Although the procedure is performed under general anaesthetic, it usually takes less than 10 minutes and is performed as a day case.

b   **False.** Although contamination with dirty water is a cause of ear infection in patients with grommets, the patient may swim so long as they are careful not to submerge the ears. Earplugs can be useful for protecting the middle ear while swimming. However, if recurrent ear infections do occur, swimming must be avoided.

c **False.** Once a grommet has been inserted, it will be expelled naturally after 10 to 12 months as a result of the migration of epithelial cells. Surgical removal is not necessary.

d **False.** The term 'permanent' may appear to be a misnomer here. Permanent grommets tend to remain in place for around 3 to 5 years.

e **False.** This is very rare, occurring in less than 2% of cases. As described above, grommets are expelled by the normal epithelial cell migration process. As a result, in the vast majority of cases no residual perforation remains.

29. a **True.** Otalgia may arise from any part of the ear, and therefore requires thorough examination of the pinna, external auditory meatus and tympanic membrane. In addition, it is important to remember that otalgia may be due to referred pain from the cranial nerves that innervate the outer and middle ear.

b **False.** Otorrhoea refers to discharge from the ear. Erythema refers to a reddened appearance. Otorrhoea is commonly accompanied by some degree of hearing loss. It is clinically important to note the odour of the discharge (offensive in chronic suppurative otitis media) and its colour (e.g. whether it is watery, purulent or bloody). Like otalgia, otorrhoea may occur due to a number of causes, from the outer ear to the middle ear, and may originate from a range of different pathologies, not just infection.

c **True.** There are three main types of investigation that should be conducted when assessing the ear, namely audiometry, vestibulometry and radiology. Audiometry encompasses pure-tone audiograms as the single most widely used subjective measure of hearing. Objective measures include oto-acoustic emissions (used mainly in neonates) and impedance audiometry (very useful for assessing middle ear disease, such as the presence of an effusion). Vestibulometry mainly assesses patients for vertigo by using a variety of techniques, from positional testing (using a series of manoeuvres) to caloric testing (the insertion of warm and cold water into the ear canal, and inspection for nystagmus). Radiology involves the imaging modalities of CT and MRI. These are very useful for investigating space-occupying lesions such as benign or malignant neoplasms.

d **False.** Tinnitus is the term used to describe the sound of ringing in the ear. It can be further differentiated into high-pitched and low-pitched tinnitus, and this distinction may yield diagnostically important clues. Otorrhoea is the term used to describe discharge from the ear.

e **False.** The word 'aural' (meaning 'ear') must not be confused with 'oral' (meaning 'mouth'). Aural drops refer to ear drops, or topical medicine that is administered in the form of drops into the ear canal.

30. a **True.**
   b **True.** It is divided into the scala vestibuli and scala media/cochlear duct by Reissner's membrane, and the basilar membrane divides the scala media and the scala tympani.
   c **False.** The scala media is filled with endolymph, which is continuously secreted by a plexus of blood vessels called the stria vascularis. It therefore has a similar composition to extracellular fluid. However, the scala vestibuli and scala tympani are filled with perilymph fluid that has a similar composition to intracellular fluid.
   d **True.**
   e **False.** The stapes is set in the oval window, which conducts sound waves along the scala vestibuli. These waves are conducted to the scala media/cochlear duct through the flexible Reissner's membrane. These waves also depress the basilar membrane, causing bulging of the round window present along the scala tympani.

31. a **True.**
   b **False.** The organ of Corti lies on the basilar membrane within the cochlear duct.
   c **True.** There are about 3500 inner hair cells (in a single row) and about 12000 outer hair cells (in three separate rows). The inner hair cells are located near the inner part of the organ of Corti. The outer hair cells are located towards the free margin of the tectorial membrane.
   d **False.** The inner hair cells provide most (around 93%) of the auditory input to the brain via nerve VIII, and the rest is provided by the outer hair cells.
   e **False.** The outer hair cells are the effector organs, and therefore receive most of the efferent input from the brainstem. These efferents modify the shape of the outer hair cells.

32. a **True.**
   b **True.**
   c **True.**

    d **False.** Maintaining good eye contact will greatly enhance communication with the patient. Not only will this help to build rapport and trust, but also it will ensure that the patient can see any facial gestures or expressions clearly.

    e **False.** Communication is not limited to speech. Facial expressions, gestures and the use of pen and paper can solve many problems in communication. Sign language is an excellent method of communicating with these patients.

33. a **True.** The chorda tympani is a branch of the facial nerve that innervates the taste receptors of the anterior third of the tongue and transmits this information to the brain. It travels through the middle ear cavity.

    b **False.** The olfactory nerve has a relatively short course and does not enter the middle ear.

    c **True.** The tympanic nerve is a branch of the glossopharyngeal nerve, and it travels through the middle ear cavity. It provides sensory innervation to the middle ear, but also carries sympathetic and parasympathetic fibres. The tympanic nerve forms a plexus in the middle ear before leaving the cavity as the lesser petrosal nerve. The lesser petrosal nerve carries the parasympathetic innervation to the parotid gland.

    d **False.** The optic nerve does not travel through the middle ear. Its course remains within the vault of the skull.

    e **False.** The trochlear nerve is responsible for adduction of the eye by supplying the innervation to the lateral rectus muscle. It does not travel through the middle ear.

34. a **True.**

    b **False.** This bone is found in the wrist, and is one of the carpal bones.

    c **True.**

    d **False.** This bone is also a carpal bone, found in the wrist.

    e **True.** Sound waves travel through the middle ear via three tiny bones. The malleus has a large area of contact with the tympanic membrane, and transfers its vibration on to the incus, which in turn is in contact with the stapes. The stapes is in contact with the inner ear, and it is within the cochlea that sound is transduced into action potentials.

35. a **True.** Rinne and Weber testing involves the use of a 512 Hz tuning fork. After striking the tuning fork against an elbow or other hard surface, it is placed initially next to the ear, and then on the mastoid process. The patient is asked in which position the tuning fork vibration was heard loudest. The same test is then repeated on the other ear. These actions make up the Rinne aspect of the test. Normally, air conduction (AC) is greater than bone conduction (BC), and is recorded simply as AC > BC. Bone conduction is greater than air conduction in conductive hearing loss (e.g. in the case of a middle ear effusion).

The Weber part of the test involves placing the tuning fork on a bone prominence anywhere in the midline of the head, usually the forehead or the top of the head. Sound should be heard equally bilaterally in a normal person. However, in conductive hearing loss, sound will be heard loudest on the affected side, and in sensorineural hearing loss, sound will be heard loudest on the better side. A false-negative result can be obtained if the contralateral ear is not masked during the test, as the tuning fork vibration may be conducted to the good ear, and hence mask sensorineural hearing loss in the affected ear. In addition, it is important to note that this question states that if air conduction (AC) is greater than bone conduction (BC) bilaterally, there may be normal hearing, because another possibility is that there may be undiagnosed mild bilateral sensorineural hearing loss!

b **True.** If the Weber test had localised to the right ear, left sensorineural hearing loss could be a possibility, especially if the right ear had not been masked with noise to avoid this.

c **False.** This situation would suggest left sensorineural hearing loss, since the sound will be detected by (and be sensed as loudest in) the cochlea with greatest function, which in this case is the right ear.

d **False.** In conductive hearing loss, Weber testing would localise to the affected ear, in this case the left ear. However, because Weber testing localises to the contralateral ear, which was also unmasked during the test, this is a false-positive result. The test should be repeated with the right ear masked by a sound generator, in order to demonstrate the true sensorineural hearing loss in the left ear.

e **True.** There may be bilateral middle ear effusions. Rinne and Weber testing can be difficult to grasp at first, and may seem intimidating, but it is an essential part of a hearing and ear examination, and all practitioners should be competent in administering it and interpreting the findings. It is a technique that is greatly improved by practice.

36. a **True.** The aetiology of skin cancer involves DNA damage due to exposure to ultraviolet light. As a result of this, skin cancers tend to occur in sun-exposed regions of the body, and the skin on the ears is at particular risk. In addition, when applying sunscreen, most people tend to forget to apply it to the ear pinna. In view of these facts, any ulceration or reddened swelling on the pinna should be viewed suspiciously until skin cancer has been ruled out.

   b **True.** A wide local excision is required in order to ensure that all of the cancer is successfully removed. This can be devastating cosmetically, and pinna reconstruction should be discussed.

   c **False.** A pearly white appearance is the characteristic sign of a basal-cell carcinoma. Squamous-cell carcinomas tend to be erythematous ulcerating lesions.

   d **False.** Antibiotics are effective against bacterial infections. The aetiology of cancer involves gene mutations, and antibiotics are of no use in treating a primary cancer

   e **False.** If left untreated, this cancer will grow and spread, and the results will be devastating. Cancers have the ability to develop their own blood supply through a process termed angiogenesis.

37. a **True.** This procedure may be performed in patients with glue ear.

   b **False.** A myomectomy is the term used to describe the surgical removal of uterine fibroids. This is a gynaecological operation, not an ENT operation.

   c **True.** This operation may be performed in patients with otosclerosis.

   d **False.** This is an abdominal operation performed in patients with appendicitis.

   e **True.** This operation may be performed in patients with mastoiditis.

38. a **True.** Deformities of the cervical spine can cause referred pain to the ear. This is more common in the elderly, and the otalgia tends to be worse on neck movement. The site of the pain may be ambiguous around the ear, or be localised to just behind the pinna. It is important to bear in mind all of the non-otological causes of otalgia, in order to prevent diagnoses being missed, as illustrated by this question.

   b **False.** There is no referred pain from the knee to the ear.

   c **True.** Inflammation of the various sinuses of the head can result in otalgia.

d **True.** Tonsillitis may cause otalgia. Post-tonsillectomy otalgia may also occur, but it usually resolves eventually.

e **False.** Epistaxis is the term used to describe a nose bleed. There is no direct relationship between epistaxis and otalgia.

39. a **True.** FBC is the abbreviation for full blood count. This investigation is particularly useful for assessing the patient's haemodynamic reserve in the event that blood loss during surgery is greater than anticipated. It also yields the white blood cell count, which is important when considering the patient's fitness for the operation, and any possible complications that may occur.

b **True.** Many operations are performed under general anaesthetic. Liver function tests are an important investigation, as many general anaesthetics are metabolised by the liver. It is therefore important to ascertain the functioning of the liver in order to administer the correct dose.

c **False.** Barium swallow is useful for imaging the upper gastrointestinal tract, but has no role in imaging of the ear.

d **False.** Technetium scanning has no role in routine imaging of the ear. It may be useful in malignant otitis externa.

e **True.** U&Es is an acronym for urea and electrolytes. This test is useful for assessing the function of the kidneys. Many of the muscle relaxants that are administered during surgery are metabolised by the kidneys, so it is important to ascertain renal function in order to adjust the dose of drugs appropriately.

40. a **False.** If the first attempt has failed to remove the foreign body, continued attempts may lead to additional trauma to the ear canal and may break up the object into several pieces that are more difficult to retrieve. It is better to have the foreign body removed conclusively under general anaesthetic.

b **False.** Batteries contain corrosive chemicals and need to be removed without delay. Plastic bodies tend to be benign and stable.

c **True.** Suction is a very effective way to remove a foreign body.

d **False.** Never push the foreign body further into the ear canal. If there is difficulty in removing the object, removal should be attempted under general anaesthetic.

e **True.** Irrigation can be used to extract the object, but should not be used for biological material, and there is also a risk of pushing the object further into the canal.

41. a **True.** Prominent ears, also referred to by the politically incorrect term 'bat ears', can cause great distress to both children and adults. They can be the source of unrelenting bullying and consequent social anxiety. They are due to the absence of antihelix development, which subsequently results in protrusion of the ears. The surgical procedure used to correct this condition is called pinnaplasty (and is also referred to as otoplasty).

   b **False.** During the first month of life, the cartilage of the ear is immature. As a result, the use of splints to alter the shape of the developing cartilage is more beneficial than surgical correction at this age. Surgical intervention should ideally be considered in children who are old enough to endure the presence of the head bandage after surgery. In practical terms, this usually involves children around the age of 5 years or older.

   c **False.** Pinnaplasty can be performed via one of two approaches, namely anterior scoring or the Mustarde technique. Both procedures have a similar prognosis, and take around 1 hour to complete. In both cases the procedures are usually performed as a day case, and the patient can be sent home with a head bandage, and followed up at an outpatient appointment to assess the outcome and remove the head bandage.

   d **True.** A head bandage is useful as it prevents the formation of a haematoma.

   e **True.** This is a serious complication and it requires urgent identification and management. If left untreated, a haematoma will cause inflammation, fibrous remodelling and subsequent distortion of the ear. Wearing a head bandage for 1 week post surgery helps to prevent the formation of a haematoma.

42. a **False.**
   b **True.**
   c **False.**
   d **True.**
   e **True.**

43. a **False.** It is most commonly due to a viral infection.
   b **True.** Vertigo can be very severe in these patients, and can prevent them from doing anything for themselves.
   c **True.** Movement makes the vertigo worse in patients with labyrinthitis.
   d **True.** In labyrinthitis, the patient's eyes may demonstrate horizontal nystagmus.

e **False.** Labyrinthitis is a clinical diagnosis made by combining a suggestive history with the related clinical signs from examination. Investigations only serve to exclude other diagnoses, and are not usually necessary.

44. a **True.** They are caused by a periosteal reaction of the tympanic bone to cold, and so are more common in swimmers, in whom cold water enters the ear canal.
     b **False.** Exostoses rarely cause any symptoms. However, they may occasionally cause a conductive hearing loss due to ear wax impaction.
     c **True.** Exostoses block the natural migration of epithelium and wax along the ear canal. This can occasionally cause a build-up of wax, and subsequent conductive hearing loss.
     d **True.** This is rarely needed. However, if symptoms persist, exostoses may be removed surgically.
     e **True.** This is due to the build-up of ear wax, as explained above.

45. a **True.**
     b **True.**
     c **True.**
     d **True.**
     e **False.** Hearing aids are available on the National Health Service, and should be offered to those patients who may benefit from using them.

46. a **True.** This question is examining knowledge of the basic constituents of a hearing aid. When explaining to a patient what a hearing aid is and how it works, this knowledge is vital. A hearing aid has three simple components, namely the input (the microphone, the process (the processor) and the output (the transmitter).
     b **False.**
     c **True.**
     d **False.**
     e **True.**

47. a **True.** Otorrhoea is a common complaint in patients with chronic suppurative otitis media.
     b **False.** Chronic suppurative otitis media has a good prognosis.
     c **True.** Cholesteatomas form due to the high pressures present within the ear in this condition.

    d **True.**

    e **True.**

48. a **False.**

    b **True.**

    c **True.**

    d **False.** It is characterised by sudden-onset pain which may persist for up to two days. Rupturing the vesicles may alleviate the pain.

    e **False.** A clinical history and simple inspection of the vesicles on the tympanic membrane via an auroscope are sufficient to diagnose the condition. Do not forget to test facial muscle strength, as bullous myringitis must be differentiated from Ramsay Hunt syndrome, which also leads to the development of vesicles in the ear canal.

49. a **True.** This question is slightly tricky in that it asks which of the patients would *not* benefit from an analogue over-the-ear hearing aid (remember to read the question carefully). A degree of hand dexterity and functionality is required by the patient, first to wear the hearing aid, and secondly to adjust the volume on it. If the patient cannot do this due to her rheumatoid hands, she is less likely to use and benefit from the device.

    b **True.** The patient must be sufficiently self-motivated to request a hearing aid, otherwise it will not be used.

    c **False.** Presbycusis is the natural deterioration of hearing with age. Since this patient has only mild to moderate hearing loss, she still has sufficient cochlear function to benefit from a hearing aid.

    d **True.** Standard analogue hearing aids merely amplify sound. If the patient has negligible cochlear function to begin with, he will receive minimal if any benefit from the device.

    e **True.** Tinnitus following loud noise is a normal phenomenon. This young man is otherwise well, with no baseline hearing loss.

50. a **False.** You would expect the patient to have otalgia (ear pain) in the case of acute otitis media. The chronic nature of the patient's symptoms and the bilateral nature of the hearing loss also exclude acute otitis media.

    b **True.** This patient may be suffering from otosclerosis, and 66% of cases are inherited. A pink but healthy eardrum is a feature of otosclerosis.

c **True.** In otosclerosis, spongy new bone replaces the normal compact bone of the stapes. This sclerosis of the foot of the stapes is responsible for the patient's symptoms. The disease is more common in young women.

d **True.** This is the first-line management of this condition. Many patients are satisfied with a simple hearing aid and so avoid the possible complications of surgical intervention.

e **True.** A stapedectomy can greatly increase hearing in the affected ear. However, there is a risk of deafness associated with this procedure, and the worst ear should be operated on first.

51. a **False.** Carbon dioxide is a normal component of air. It is not relevant to the aetiology of otitis externa.

b **False.** Asbestos has severe consequences for the lungs if inhaled, but it does not cause otitis externa.

c **True.** Herpes simplex and herpes zoster give rise to vesiculation of the tympanic membrane and ear canal.

d **True.** Fungi (e.g. *Candida albicans*) may give rise to otitis externa.

e **True.** Bacterial infection is commonly associated with otitis externa.

52. a **True.** Meningitis can result in progressive sensorineural hearing loss.

b **True.** Chemotherapeutic agents may damage the hair cells in the inner ear that are responsible for transducing sound waves into action potentials.

c **False.** This abnormal growth occurs in the middle ear and causes a conductive hearing loss, not a sensorineural hearing loss. It usually presents unilaterally, and can cause both deafness and vertigo.

d **True.** Neonatal hypoxia can cause bilateral sensorineural hearing loss.

e **False.** This is an infection of the middle ear, and it presents with a conductive hearing loss, not a sensorineural hearing loss.

53. a **True.** Basal-cell cancers tend to appear as a raised pearly white lesion on inflamed surrounding tissue.

b **False.** The question is referring to localised (non-metastatic) basal-cell carcinoma. Wide local excision is the accepted treatment for this condition. The excised tissue may then be sent for further histological analysis.

c **False.** Squamous-cell carcinomas are the most likely to metastasise, not basal-cell carcinomas.

d **False.** This best describes squamous-cell carcinoma. Basal-cell cancers tend to appear as raised pearly white lesions on inflamed surrounding tissue.

e **True.** This is to ensure that none of the cancer is left behind. Since these cancers may be located on the pinna of the ear, a wide local excision can be devastating cosmetically. Skin grafts and cosmetic remodelling are required to reconstruct the pinna as best as possible.

54. a **False.** Coughing is a reflex to clear the airway. The Eustachian tube has no role in this process.

b **False.** Cerumen is another name for ear wax. Ear wax leaves the outer ear by the process of epithelial migration. The Eustachian tube connects the nasopharynx with the middle ear, not the outer ear.

c **True.** This helps to prevent infection occurring in the middle ear.

d **False.** Sneezing is also a reflex to help to clear the airway. The Eustachian tube has no role in this process.

e **True.** This is an important role of the Eustachian tube, and blockage can result in tympanic perforation due to the build-up of excess pressure.

55. a **False.** There is no link between mastoiditis and lung cancer.

b **True.** The infection of mastoiditis can enter the cranial cavity by erosion. Mastoiditis can occur as a complication of otitis media. It is a potentially fatal condition, and should be treated rapidly in order to prevent devastating complications.

c **False.** There is no link between mastoiditis and irritable bowel syndrome.

d **True.** The infection can destroy the bone.

e **False.** Mastoiditis does not cause laryngeal stenosis.

56. a **False.** If left untreated, mastoiditis can cause serious complications. It must be treated aggressively.

b **True.** These are given to control the infection. A myringotomy may also help to drain an effusion if the middle ear is the source of the infection.

c **True.** This involves surgically removing the infected part of the mastoid bone.

d **False.** In most cases, defibrillation is reserved for cardiac arrest and certain cardiac arrhythmias. It has no place in the treatment of mastoiditis.

e **False.** The use of a nasal tampon is reserved for epistaxis. This does not occur in mastoiditis, and therefore a nasal tampon is not needed.

57. a **False.** Parotitis describes infection of the parotid gland. It is not in any way related to hearing loss.
    b **True.** Certain medications can result in sensorineural hearing loss.
    c **True.** Dominant progressive hearing loss (DPHL) is an inherited condition which can affect young people, and that results in a progressive sensorineural hearing loss. A detailed family history of hearing loss should be taken in order to elucidate this diagnosis.
    d **False.** Skull fractures can result in a sudden hearing loss, not a progressive hearing loss.
    e **True.** Exposure to loud noise over a longer period of time is damaging to hearing. It is a cause of progressive degeneration of hearing.

58. a **True.** This is especially true in cases where children are born into families where neither parent learns to use sign language to communicate. With supportive home environments and the use of sign language by all members of the family, there is no social delay.
    b **False.** Difficulty swallowing is not encountered by a child with isolated pre-lingual deafness.
    c **True.** This is particularly true for children who have not learned to use sign language, or who are put in situations where no one else understands sign language.
    d **False.** Motor development is unaffected by pre-lingual deafness. However, social development may become greatly delayed.
    e **True.** These emotions stem from the frustration that arises due to communication barriers. These children may vent their agitation in a number of ways, and the key to addressing these problems is to establish a common platform of communication between all those concerned (the child, their parents and their teachers). This may take the form of teaching and learning sign language. Special schools for deaf children allow a feeling of acceptance and belonging to develop, and greatly improve the self-confidence and behaviour of pre-lingual deaf children.

59. a **False.** Sensorineural hearing loss is caused by a neuronal defect, and no amount of shouting will result in better conduction of

sound at the frequencies in which the patient is deficient.

b **False.** Patients lip-read best when you are speaking at normal speed. By slowing down your speech, you will be distorting and emphasising words in an abnormal way compared with normal speech. Make sure that you do not mask your lips with your hands or turn away as you speak, as this may hinder the patient's ability to lip-read and understand you.

c **True.** Patients with sensorineural hearing loss benefit greatly from seeing the facial expressions and hand gestures of the person to whom they are speaking. Lip-reading may also fill in gaps of communication. You should speak at your normal speed and level of speech.

d **True.** Sign language interpreters are invaluable when communicating with an individual who has been deaf for some time and has learned how to use sign language. Remember that in cases of sudden deafness, patients may not understand sign language.

e **True.** Diagrams are an excellent way of explaining a concept to both hearing and deaf people.

60. a **True.** Patients who acquire hearing loss later in life are able to read and understand written information. This is very useful during a consultation, as questions and answers can be written down on a piece of paper.

b **False.** The patient must be your primary concern, and time spent ensuring that you are communicating with them is invaluable. It is the patient who must live with any diagnosis that is made, and the patient who must adhere to any treatment regime, not the relative. Spending additional time on communicating with the patient will be beneficial in establishing a stronger rapport, therapeutic relationship and mutual trust. Always remember that just because a patient has hearing loss this does not mean that they lack capacity. You should always check whether the patient actually consents to the person who is accompanying them remaining in the consultation.

c **False.** Most patients with sudden hearing loss do not understand sign language, and the sudden nature of their condition means that they have not had time to learn it.

d **False.** Sensorineural hearing loss is caused by a neuronal defect, and no amount of shouting will result in better conduction of sound at the frequencies in which the patient is deficient.

e **False.** If this policy is always followed, these patients will continually fall through the gaps. The skilled physician can negotiate the communication difficulties and still finish on time, but it is important to remember that these patients may well require additional time to communicate. Prior planning is very effective in this situation. For example, a double appointment can be helpful in primary care, and in secondary care these patients can be placed near the end of the clinic to prevent other patients being inconvenienced by having to wait too long.

61. a **False.** This may be otitis media, and it therefore carries a very good prognosis.
b **True.** Bilateral hearing loss has a poor prognosis.
c **True.** Unfortunately, the presence of vertigo implies a more serious and poorer outcome in terms of hearing.
d **True.** Sudden hearing loss in children has a poorer prognosis than that in adults.
e **True.** Initial severe hearing loss indicates a poor prognosis.

62. a **True.** It is usually advised that cerumenolytic ear drops should be taken three times a day up to 5 days before syringing. Cerumenolytic agents range from simple olive oil to carbamide peroxide. These agents help to soften the wax so that it can be easily removed by syringing.
b **False.** This is below the freezing point of water, and will probably turn to ice in the syringe! Lukewarm water is required at around 37–38°C in order to successfully break up the wax. Cold water will cause vertigo.
c **False.** The syringe should be aimed upwards and backwards in the ear canal in order to minimise the risk of eardrum perforation. Aiming downwards and forwards will pose a real risk of damage to the tympanic membrane.
d **True.** Lukewarm water is required to successfully break up and remove the cerumen (ear wax) without causing unwanted side-effects. Colder temperatures result in the patient complaining of the unpleasant sensation of vertigo.
e **True.** This is to minimise the risk of eardrum perforation. After syringing, the head should be lowered on the side that has been syringed in order to allow the water and ear wax to drain out. The procedure is then repeated if required.

63. a **True.** By tilting the head or by placing a hand over the affected ear while washing, water can be prevented from entering the ear canal and exacerbating the otitis externa.

b **True.** Swimming in dirty water may allow pathogens to enter the ear canal and worsen the infection.

c **False.** The patient should be advised to avoid letting water enter the ear canal. A cotton ball covered with petroleum jelly is a very effective plug which can be used to cover the ear canal. It should not be inserted into the ear canal, but just over it to prevent water entering it while washing.

d **False.** There is no link between cranberry juice and otitis externa (although cranberry juice can be advised for patients with urinary tract infections).

e **True.** The best advice to give this patient would be not to insert anything into the external ear. The localised damage caused by cotton buds or other objects can result in another bout of otitis externa.

64. a **False.** The ear must be kept dry in order to avoid exacerbating the otitis externa.

b **True.** Analgesics (painkillers) such as paracetamol are very useful for treating the otalgia (ear pain) caused by otitis externa.

c **False.** Listening to loud music has no effect on otitis externa.

d **True.** Antibiotics are used in severe cases. However, some cases of otitis externa are caused by fungal infections.

e **True.** These include keeping the ear canal dry while washing, avoiding swimming in dirty water, and avoiding inserting cotton buds or any other objects into the ear canal.

65. a **True.** Not all cases of otitis externa are caused by bacteria. *Aspergillus* and *Candida* are the most common species of fungi that cause otitis externa.

b **True.** This pathogen is responsible for over a third of all cases of otitis externa. *Staphylococcus aureus* and *Pseudomonas aeruginosa* are the most common bacterial causes of otitis externa.

c **False.** Rhinovirus is one of the viruses responsible for the common cold and symptoms such as coryza, but it is not a direct cause of otitis externa.

d **True.** As stated above, *Staphylococcus aureus* and *Pseudomonas aeruginosa* are the most common bacterial causes of otitis externa.

e **True.** As explained above, this is a fungal cause of otitis externa.

66. a **True.** Malignant otitis externa is otherwise known as necrotising otitis externa. It occurs in patients who are immunocompromised. HIV patients fall into this category, and are at risk of a number of other infections.

b **True.** Excessive steroid use suppresses the immune system.

c **True.** Long-term uncontrolled diabetes may be regarded as an immunocompromised state, and therefore these patients are susceptible to malignant otitis media.

d **True.** Chemotherapy destroys all rapidly dividing cells and disrupts the immune system.

e **True.** Natural defences wear down with increasing age, and a painful itchy ear with a foul-smelling discharge in an elderly patient should warn you of possible malignant otitis media.

67. a **True.** The patient may complain of a continual itch arising from the ear canal. They must be carefully advised not to insert any object (e.g. a cotton bud) into the ear.

b **True.** A foul-smelling yellow discharge may appear from the affected ear.

c **False.** Coughing is not a feature of malignant otitis media.

d **True.** Hearing loss is a common complaint in patients with malignant otitis media.

e **True.** Otalgia (ear pain) is a common feature of malignant otitis media, with or without a high temperature.

68. a **False.** Ménière's disease would present with the classic combination of vertigo, tinnitus and sensorineural hearing loss. However, this patient does not complain of these symptoms.

b **False.** Labyrinthitis commonly presents with dizziness, and usually follows an upper respiratory tract infection. There is no such history in this case.

c **False.** Benign paroxysmal positional vertigo presents with brief episodes of vertigo. On examination, nystagmus and vertigo can be elicited by the Dix–Hallpike manoeuvre. This was negative in this patient.

d **False.** This is an abnormal connection between the middle and inner ear, which can be congenital or traumatic. The result is vertigo and hearing loss.

e **True.** This patient is suffering from the classic symptoms of vertebrobasilar insufficiency. The blood flow to the anterior and posterior inferior cerebellar arteries is restricted due to compression of the vertebral artery on neck extension. It is usually caused by bony spurs or abnormalities of the cervical spine that occur with increasing age. It is important to remember that not all patients who attend an ENT clinic will have problems with the ear, nose or throat. Keeping in mind other possibilities is the only way you can diagnose conditions that have been missed by others.

69. a **False.** Metronidazole will not destroy the likely pathogens involved in meningitis. This child requires a third-generation cephalosporin such as ceftriaxone. Cefotaxime is used in adults.

    b **True.** Meningitis is a serious complication of acute otitis media, and must be recognised and treated early.

    c **False.** The child may die if you take this course of action. He requires urgent antibiotics and admission to hospital. He will require a spinal tap for cerebrospinal fluid analysis when he is more stable.

    d **True.** Nothing should delay this course of action.

    e **False.** Meningitis is treated with antibiotics. Nothing should delay treatment. Recognition is key, and delay in diagnosing the condition is often the main cause of mortality.

70. a **False.** *Staphylococcus* is not a congenital infection that causes hearing loss. Not all cases of deafness are genetic or acquired in adulthood. Congenital infections such as syphilis, rubella and cytomegalovirus are important causes of deafness. Most are screened for in the mother by routine pregnancy blood tests, such as the TORCH investigations.

    b **True.** Deafness caused by syphilis may not be apparent immediately, and may only start to develop in the teenage years or even later.

    c **True.** Rubella is a devastating congenital infection that causes, among other things, profound sensorineural hearing loss.

    d **False.** Candida is not a congenital infection that causes hearing loss.

    e **True.** Cytomegalovirus does not cause hearing loss in all infected children, but among those who are affected the deafness can worsen with time.

71. a **False.** This question examines understanding of the relevant basic anatomy. The submandibular salivary gland is located under the chin. The parotid gland is located just in front of the ear and runs deep to the cheek. As a result, in acute bacterial parotitis there is swelling of the cheek, not under the chin.

    b **False.** There is no link between acute bacterial parotitis and acute otitis externa.

c **True.** The parotid gland is located just in front of the ear and runs deep to the cheek.

d **False.** Acute bacterial parotitis is a bacterial infection of the parotid salivary gland. Nasal decongestants can be useful in sinusitis but are of no use in this condition. Antibiotics are required to treat the infection.

e **True.** Chewing exacerbates the pain in acute bacterial parotitis.

72. a **True.**

b **True.** Patients complain of a discharge from the affected ear.

c **False.** Patients may have a conductive hearing loss, not a sensorineural hearing loss.

d **True.** If there was no tympanic membrane perforation, there would be no otorrhoea (discharge from the ear), and therefore the diagnosis of CSOM could not apply. If the tympanic membrane is intact and a middle ear effusion is present, the diagnosis of serous otitis media can be made.

e **False.** The diagnosis of chronic suppurative otitis media is only made if the symptoms of otorrhoea and conductive hearing loss last for longer than 6 months, not 2 weeks.

73. a **False.** This is a difficult question, and it examines knowledge of the nomenclature used to classify cases of chronic suppurative otitis media (CSOM). The initial classification of CSOM depends on the presence or absence of a cholesteatoma. Cholesteatomas are abnormal growths of squamous epithelium. CSOM with cholesteatoma is described as 'unsafe', and that without cholesteatoma is classified as 'safe.' Safe CSOM (without cholesteatomas) is then further divided into CSOM with infection ('active' type) and CSOM without infection ('inactive' type). The relevance of categorising CSOM in this way becomes apparent when discussing management. The answer to this first question is that CSOM with cholesteatoma is regarded as an 'unsafe' type, not an 'active' type (which is reserved for cases of CSOM with no cholesteatoma, but with infection also present).

b **False.** The term 'radioactive' is not used to describe CSOM. This case would be described as 'unsafe active.'

c **False.** This is described as 'active', as explained above.

d **False.** This is described as 'unsafe', as explained above.

e **False.** This is described as 'inactive', as explained above.

74. a **True.** Fluid in the middle ear may cause a conductive hearing loss.

   b **True.** The Eustachian tube drains fluid from the middle ear. If it is blocked, fluid and consequently pressure builds up here.

   c **True.** In children, the horizontal Eustachian tube can exacerbate any blockage. As the child grows, the Eustachian tube becomes more oblique. As a result it is less likely to become blocked, and symptoms may improve or disappear with age.

   d **False.** Serous otitis media by definition does not result in tympanic membrane perforation.

   e **True.** Allergy is a cause of serous otitis media. Therefore antihistamines may help to alleviate some of the symptoms of this condition.

75. a **True.** As a child develops, the Eustachian tube changes to adopt the adult configuration. The immature Eustachian tube in children is more horizontal than that in adults. As the child grows, the tube becomes more oblique until it reaches its final adult position. It is this anatomical difference that is responsible for the higher rates of middle ear infections in children compared with the adult population.

   b **True.** The Eustachian tube opens between the adenoid tissues. When this tissue hypertrophies, it can easily block off the Eustachian tube.

   c **False.** An enlarged tongue will not block the Eustachian tubes, which open into the nasopharynx.

   d **True.** Infection sparks an inflammatory response with mucosal swelling. Mucosal swelling can also occur in response to allergens. It is this swelling that is responsible for blocking the Eustachian tube. As a result, antibiotics or antihistamines may be used to treat the consequences of Eustachian tube blockage.

   e **False.** Acute otitis externa is an infection of the outer ear. It cannot cause Eustachian tube blockage.

76. a **False.** Cholesteatoma is not a neoplasm or tumour. It is the abnormal destructive growth of normal squamous epithelium within the middle ear, and can be either congenital or acquired. If it is left untreated it will continue to grow and cause local damage.

   b **False.** If left untreated, it will continue to grow and destroy local structures. For this reason it should be treated.

   c **False.** Cholesteatomas consist of squamous epithelium.

d **False.** Cholesteatomas are not neoplasms or tumours and do not metastasise. However, they can be very destructive when they grow into the inner ear and destroy bone.

e **False.** Surgical intervention is the only treatment for cholesteatoma. Antibiotics and conservative measures to keep the ear clean will not prevent growth of the cholesteatoma.

77. a **True.** Dizziness ensues when the cholesteatoma has started to invade the inner ear.

b **True.** Hearing loss results from physical conductive hearing loss, cerumen impaction, destruction of the ossicles and later destruction of the cochlea as the cholesteatoma invades the inner ear.

c **False.** There is no relationship between cholesteatoma and the thyroid gland.

d **True.** A cholesteatoma can grow and erode the facial nerve, resulting in a facial paralysis.

e **True.** The cholesteatoma does not only erode structures along the course of the ear canal, but will also erode upwards, and can cause infection to seed in the layers covering the brain (meningitis). There is also a possibility of brain abscess formation.

78. a **False.** Laryngeal cancer is not an indication for the insertion of a grommet.

b **True.** Grommets help to aerate or ventilate the middle ear.

c **False.** Grommets cannot relieve the symptoms of parotitis.

d **False.** Grommets are not used to treat adenoid hypertrophy. If the adenoids are causing symptoms by blocking the Eustachian tube, they can be surgically removed.

e **True.** If a patient is experiencing recurrent episodes of otitis media or has had complications due to recurrent otitis media (e.g. mastoiditis), the insertion of a grommet is indicated.

79. a **True.**

b **False.** They consist of one large kinocilium and 50–150 stereocilia.

c **False.** The tip of the stereocilium is bathed in endolymph, which has a high potassium concentration (150 mM) and a very low sodium concentration (1 mM).

d **False.** The body of the hair cell is bathed in perilymph, which has a low potassium concentration (7 mM) and a high sodium concentration (140 mM).

e **False.** Mechanical deformation against the kinocilium (the tallest cilium) closes the potassium channels, whereas deformation towards the kinocilium opens the potassium channels. The cilia that are bent in the direction of the kinocilium cause an inward potassium current flow in the cell, resulting in its depolarisation and thus opening the voltage-gated calcium channels and allowing the release of neurotransmitter (acetylcholine) on to afferent nerve fibres.

80. a **True.**
    b **False.** The stapes ossicle develops from the second pharyngeal arch.
    c **True.**
    d **False.** The thyroid cartilage is not located in the middle ear, and is in fact derived from the fourth pharyngeal arch.
    e **False.** The thymus is not located in the middle ear, and is in fact derived from the third pharyngeal arch.

81. a **False.** The term microtia refers to small ears. Macrotia refers to large ears.
    b **False.** Anotia is the term used to describe an absent ear.
    c **True.** Synotia is the term used to describe ears that are too close together anteriorly.
    d **True.** Melotia is the term used to describe defective developmental ascent of the ear and its subsequent presence at the level of the cheek.
    e **False.** Macroglossia is the term used to describe a large tongue. Macrotia is the term used to describe large ears.

82. a **True.** Vertigo is often described as a spinning sensation, but it is in fact a hallucination of motion that can be in any direction.
    b **False.** See above.
    c **False.** The triad of symptoms that make up Ménière's disease consists of vertigo, tinnitus and hearing loss.
    d **True.** Vertigo that is due to a condition called benign paroxysmal positional vertigo (BPPV) may be relieved by the Epley manoeuvre. In this condition, calcium crystals or otoconia are displaced from their normal positions within the inner ear to lie elsewhere, causing abnormal endolymph fluid displacement on motion and thus a sensation of vertigo. The head and neck are turned in various directions during the Epley manoeuvre in order to return the displaced otoconia to their original position.

e **True.** This is a major cause of pathological imbalance, and often the cause of natural imbalance in older people. Coordinated balance is mediated by ocular, inner ear and proprioceptive inputs that are interpreted and acted upon by the cerebellum and cerebral cortex. If the signals from these three main inputs are at odds with each other, the brain makes an attempt to interpret what it thinks is right, but the final result is sometimes a feeling of imbalance or vertigo. Older people often have age-related degeneration of the eyes, ears or joints, and so as a result of mismatched sensory inputs from these different areas balance can sometimes naturally deteriorate as one gets older. Mismatched sensory inputs are also responsible for sea sickness, car sickness and alcohol-induced imbalance.

83. a **False.** The ear is a self-cleansing organ, and natural epithelial migration removes wax and debris.
    b **False.** Nothing should be inserted into the ear canal except by a doctor or nurse when appropriate.
    c **True.**
    d **True.** The consistency in Africans and Europeans tends to be more moist and oily, whereas in Asians it tends to be more dry and flaky.
    e **True.**

The nose

Questions

1. With regard to epistaxis (bleeding from the nose), which of the following statements are true?
   a It is most commonly idiopathic in origin.
   b It is most common in children and middle-aged people.
   c It commonly originates from Little's area in the posterior aspect of the nasal septum.
   d After the nose has been packed, anterior septal bleeds can be cauterised using a silver nitrate stick.
   e It can be a cause of severe shock.

2. The following are symptoms of allergic rhinitis:
   a Sneezing.
   b Epistaxis.
   c Rhinorrhoea.
   d Cough.
   e A blocked nose.

3. Management of allergic rhinitis may involve the following:
   a Use of antihistamine medication.
   b Nasal decongestants.
   c Removal of allergens.
   d Surgical ligation of the olfactory nerve.
   e Desensitisation therapy.

4. Common allergens in allergic rhinitis include the following:
   a Pollen.
   b Cat.
   c Nuts.
   d Plastic.
   e Dust mite.

5. Regarding allergic rhinitis, which of the following statements are true?
   a It is synonymous with intrinsic rhinitis.
   b Continuous use of nasal decongestant therapy may cause rhinitis medicamentosa.
   c It is a type 1 hypersensitivity reaction.
   d It is an IgA-mediated reaction.
   e It is not linked to atopic conditions.

6. Nasal polyps may present with the following symptoms:
   a Chronic sinusitis.
   b Increasing nasal obstruction.
   c A neck lump.
   d Hypersalivation.
   e Rhinorrhoea.

7. The following are possible causes of nasal polyps:
   a Chronic sinusitis.
   b Rhinitis.
   c Bronchiectasis.
   d Bowel cancer.
   e Cystic fibrosis.

8. Management options for nasal polyps include the following:
   a Continuous high-level sympathomimetic nasal decongestants.
   b Radiotherapy.
   c Chemotherapy.
   d Nasal steroids.
   e Surgical removal.

9. Regarding a foreign body in the nose, which of the following statements are true?
   a If several unsuccessful attempts have been made to remove the foreign body, the examiner must persevere.
   b An inorganic foreign body will disintegrate over time, and requires no further treatment.
   c A foreign body may present with nasal discharge.
   d Foreign bodies in the nose are more common in the elderly.
   e They are more common in Asians.

10. Viruses that may cause the common cold include the following:
   a Rhinovirus.
   b *E. coli.*
   c Adenovirus.
   d Epstein–Barr virus.
   e Human papillomavirus.

11. The following may be symptoms of the common cold:
   a Rhinorrhoea.
   b Diarrhoea.
   c Sneezing.
   d Haematemesis.
   e Nasal congestion.

12. The following may be involved in management of the common cold:
   a Topical decongestants.
   b Steam inhalation.
   c Vigorous activity to 'shake it off.'
   d Paracetamol for mild fever or joint pain.
   e Antibiotics.

13. In a patient who presents with sinusitis, the following symptoms indicate a potentially serious complication:
   a Periorbital swelling or redness.
   b Sudden abnormal behaviour or change in personality.
   c Severe headache.
   d Rhinorrhoea.
   e Cranial nerve palsies.

14. The following granulomatous diseases affect the nose:
   a Syphilis.
   b Systemic lupus erythematosus (SLE).
   c Wegener's granulomatosis.
   d Osteoarthritis.
   e Sarcoidosis.

15. The following may be causes of nasal septal perforation:
    a   Recurrent nasal cocaine use.
    b   Trauma.
    c   Sneezing.
    d   Intravenous injection of heroin.
    e   Syphilis.

16. The following are causes of nasal septal deviation:
    a   Vocal cord polyp.
    b   Congenital.
    c   Chronic cough.
    d   Recurrent sneezing.
    e   Trauma.

17. Regarding antrochoanal polyps, the following statements are true:
    a   They appear similar to nasal polyps.
    b   They arise from within the nose.
    c   They usually appear unilaterally, in one nostril only.
    d   They can be treated with steroid nasal sprays.
    e   They require surgical intervention.

18. Regarding periorbital cellulitis, the following statements are true:
    a   It may be a complication of ethmoidal sinusitis.
    b   Input from an ophthalmologist should be sought.
    c   It may follow an upper respiratory tract infection.
    d   It requires intravenous broad-spectrum antibiotics.
    e   It may present with pain around the eye.

19. A man presents to A&E with cheek swelling. As the first person to see him, you should keep the following diagnoses in mind:
    a   Facial bone fracture.
    b   Severe dental decay.
    c   Sinus malignancy.
    d   Zenker's diverticulum.
    e   Tympanic membrane perforation.

20. A 26-year-old man sustained a nasal fracture 12 days ago during a pub fight. He has come into theatre today for nasal manipulation to straighten his nose under general anaesthetic. You have been asked to take consent from him for the procedure. Which of the following statements are true?
    a   He has come too late and nothing can be done so long after the initial trauma.
    b   The nose may not be restored to its previous appearance.
    c   The procedure will cure any accompanying septal deviation.
    d   He may require an external splint.
    e   The procedure may result in bleeding.

21. A young man has come in for his scheduled adenoidectomy. You have been asked to consent him. The following are possible complications of which he should be made aware:
    a   Once removed, the adenoid tissue may re-grow, but not to the symptomatic size.
    b   He will experience recurrent lower respiratory tract infections.
    c   He may experience excessive bleeding.
    d   The procedure is performed through the mouth, so he will have no visible scars.
    e   He may have some nasopharyngeal regurgitation.

22. A young man has come to see you to discuss the management of his septal deviation, which is causing nasal obstruction. Regarding septoplasty, which of the following statements are true?
    a   Septal perforation may occur.
    b   Septal haematoma may occur.
    c   It may not cure his symptoms.
    d   Acute nasal obstruction may occur.
    e   Bleeding can occur.

23. Wegener's granulomatosis refers to a triad that includes the following features:
    a   Glomerulonephritis.
    b   Bowel cancer.
    c   Respiratory tract granulomas.
    d   Osteoporosis.
    e   Vasculitis.

24. The following symptoms or signs will raise the suspicion of a cancer of the maxillary antrum:
a Change in bowel habit.
b Palpitations.
c Unilateral nasal obstruction.
d Back pain.
e Bloody nasal discharge.

25. A patient presents to you in A&E following a fight earlier in the evening. Which of the following statements about septal haematoma are true?
a It usually occurs after trauma to the nose.
b It may become infected and cause a septal abscess.
c It should be left alone as it will resolve spontaneously.
d If left untreated it could cause a saddle nose.
e It may cause a nasal obstruction.

26. The following are possible causes of anosmia:
a Nasal polyps.
b Acute otitis media.
c Nasal cocaine use.
d Parotid gland cancer.
e Olfactory bulb tumours.

27. A 32-year-old man attends A&E following a fight. He complains of anosmia and a unilateral transparent watery nasal discharge. You have been asked to see him, and you note a multitude of traumatic bruises on his face and body. Which of the following statements are true about this patient?
a He is suffering from incidental rhinorrhoea.
b The discharge is due to a nasal polyp.
c He has a fracture in the region of the pterion.
d He is leaking cerebrospinal fluid.
e He has a fracture of the anterior fossa/cribriform plate.

28. Acute bacterial sinusitis may be caused by the following:
a *Moraxella catarrhalis.*
b Adenovirus.
c *Streptococcus pneumoniae.*
d *E. coli.*
e *Haemophilus influenzae.*

29. During a ward round, the consultant explains to you that the patient you are seeing has chronic inflammatory sinusitis. He asks you to name the triad of conditions for this diagnosis. The following are part of the triad:
    a Nasal polyps.
    b Diarrhoea.
    c NSAID sensitivity.
    d Asthma.
    e Septic arthritis.

30. A patient with cystic fibrosis comes to see you about his sinusitis. The following statements about this patient are true:
    a Thick mucus production is responsible for sinusitis.
    b He is more likely to have HIV.
    c Nasal polyps may also contribute to sinusitis.
    d Mucolytics may be used.
    e He is more likely to have *Pseudomonas aeruginosa* in his mucus.

31. The following pathogens may be isolated from an HIV patient with sinusitis:
    a Mycobacterium.
    b *Pneumocystis carinii.*
    c Human papillomavirus.
    d Epstein–Barr virus.
    e *Pseudomonas* species.

32. The following viruses may cause rhinitis:
    a Respiratory syncytial virus.
    b *Staphylococcus aureus.*
    c *Haemophilus influenzae.*
    d Human papillomavirus.
    e Rhinovirus.

33. The following are differential diagnoses for a patient presenting with rhinitis:
    a Nasal polyps.
    b Urinary tract infection.
    c Allergic rhinitis.
    d Vasomotor rhinitis.
    e Infectious rhinitis.

34. Regarding the embryology of the nose, the following statements are true:
a The nose partly develops from neural crest cells.
b The nose begins to develop by week 4 of gestation.
c The nose begins to develop by week 20 of gestation.
d The nasal conchi form at 4 weeks' gestation.
e The nasal placodes are of ectodermal origin.

35. The following may be features of acute sinusitis:
a Facial pain that is worse on coughing.
b Vomiting.
c Pain around the maxillary region.
d Nasal obstruction.
e A recent upper respiratory tract infection.

36. Chronic rhinitis can result in turbinate hypertrophy, further exacerbating the nasal obstruction. The following techniques are used to treat turbinate hypertrophy:
a Submucosal diathermy.
b Tonsillectomy.
c Myringectomy.
d Surgical turbinate trimming.
e Nasal septal perforation.

37. The following may be signs or symptoms of a retained nasal foreign body:
a Unilateral nasal discharge.
b Facial pain.
c Difficulty breathing through the nose.
d Cataract formation.
e Chvostek's sign.

38. Regarding nasal septal haematoma, the following statements are true:
a Nasal deformity occurs.
b The nasal septum may appear asymmetrical.
c The septal haematoma usually forms within 5 minutes of nasal trauma.
d A swelling may be felt inside the nose along the nasal septum.
e It should be left alone as it will resolve spontaneously.

39. The following may be complications of a septal haematoma:
- a Saddle nose formation.
- b Septal perforation.
- c Dysphagia.
- d Septal abscess formation.
- e Ventricular fibrillation.

40. The following may be complications of sinusitis:
- a Laryngeal cancer.
- b Periorbital sinusitis.
- c Dysuria.
- d Otosclerosis.
- e Frontal lobe abscess.

41. The following statements about epiphora are true:
- a Epiphora is the term used to describe dry eyes.
- b It can be treated by eye drops.
- c Epiphora is the term used to describe excessive tear production.
- d It has a poor prognosis.
- e It may be treated by endoscopic dacryocystorhinostomy (DCR).

42. Which of the following statements about endoscopic dacryocystorhinostomy (DCR) in the treatment of epiphora are true?
- a It involves making an incision along the length of the nose.
- b It results in a large facial scar.
- c It requires a hospital stay of 7–10 days after the procedure.
- d It is a day-case procedure.
- e It can be performed under spinal block anaesthesia.

43. Complications and problems of endoscopic dacryocystorhinostomy (DCR) in the treatment of epiphora include the following:
- a A blocked nose.
- b Bleeding.
- c Coughing.
- d Anosmia.
- e Difficulty removing the drainage device.

44. Which of the following statements about the middle meatus within the nasal cavity are true?
a The maxillary sinus drains into the middle meatus.
b The anterior ethmoid sinus drains into the middle meatus.
c The sphenoethmoidal sinus drains into the middle meatus.
d The middle meatus contains the opening of the nasolacrimal duct.
e The posterior ethmoid sinus drains into the middle meatus.

45. Regarding the nasal conchae, which of the following statements are true?
a There are four conchae.
b The conchae protrude from the nasal septum medially.
c There are two meatuses.
d They help to cool the inspired air.
e They help to dry the inspired air.

46. Which of the following statements about the sense of smell are true?
a The sense of smell is mediated by the oculomotor nerve.
b Anosmia describes a heightened sense of smell.
c The sense of smell is mediated by the facial nerve.
d The sense of smell may be lost in cases of nasal congestion.
e Smell is detected via a G-protein cascade mechanism.

47. Which of the following statements about the histology of the nasal mucosa are true?
a The superficial layer mainly consists of squamous cells.
b Goblet cells are present.
c Columnar cells are ciliated.
d It is composed of astrocytes.
e It has an abundant supply of blood in the lamina propria layer.

48. Regarding the neural innervation of the nose, which of the following statements are true?
a Sensation to the skin overlying the nose is innervated by the trigeminal nerve.
b The nasal septum is innervated by the cochlear nerve.
c The optic nerve transmits the sense of smell.
d The olfactory nerve axons traverse the cribriform plate.
e The cribriform plate is formed from the ethmoid bone.

49. Factors that may exacerbate epistaxis include the following:
    a Von Willebrand disease.
    b Warfarin.
    c Vitamin K deficiency.
    d Thalassaemia.
    e Haemophilia.

50. Regarding rhinoplasty, which of the following statements are true?
    a It is synonymous with septoplasty.
    b It can be performed in order to improve function.
    c It refers to reconstruction of the ear.
    d It may result in periorbital bruising.
    e It can be performed for cosmetic reasons.

51. Which of the following statements about the nasal meatuses are true?
    a The superior meatus is located between the nasal roof and the superior concha.
    b The frontal sinus drains into the superior meatus.
    c The nasolacrimal duct opens into the inferior meatus.
    d The inferior meatus is located between the middle and inferior conchae.
    e Tears from the lacrimal sac enter the superior meatus.

52. The following bacteria may be found in the normal nasal flora:
    a *Staphylococcus epidermidis.*
    b *E. coli.*
    c *Staphylococcus aureus.*
    d *Haemophilus influenzae.*
    e *Helicobacter pylori.*

53. The following bacteria found in the nasal flora can be pathogenic:
    a *Haemophilus influenzae.*
    b *Chlamydia trachomatis.*
    c *Staphylococcus epidermidis.*
    d *Legionella pneumophila.*
    e *Streptococcus pneumoniae.*

54. Regarding sinusitis in children, which of the following statements are true?
    a The sphenoid sinus is most affected.
    b The child may have a fever.
    c It is most commonly caused by *Helicobacter pylori*.
    d It may be treated with antibiotics.
    e It tends to present with vomiting.

55. With regard to nasal obstruction, which of the following statements are true?
    a The narrowest part of the nose is at the front.
    b Deviated nasal septae can be present without any history of trauma.
    c People with hayfever often complain of the blockage shifting from one side of the nose to the other at different times.
    d Congenital obstruction of the posterior choani needs to be ruled out in a neonate with breathing difficulties.
    e Adenoidal hypertrophy is a common cause in young children.

The nose

Answers

1. a **True.** Although trauma, neoplasm, hypertension and coagulation disorders (as well as some rarer causes, such as Osler–Weber–Rendu syndrome) all play a role in epistaxis, 80% of nosebleeds are idiopathic in nature.

   b **False.** Epistaxis commonly occurs in the young (children and young people, and in the elderly (those over 70 years of age), but not in the middle-aged.

   c **False.** Epistaxis most commonly originates from Little's area. However, the latter is located in the *anterior* aspect of the septum, not the posterior aspect. Little's area is the anastomosis of four main arteries, namely the anterior ethmoidal artery, the sphenopalatine artery, the greater palatine artery, and the septal branch of the superior labial artery.

   d **True.** Never forget to assess Airways, Breathing and Circulation initially. Put on protective eyewear, gown and gloves. If the patient is not acutely shocked, the management of epistaxis from anterior septal bleeds involves tilting the head forward and applying pressure to Little's area using your fingers to try to reduce bleeding for over 10 minutes. After blowing the nose, it should be filled with a ribbon gauze drenched in 4% lidocaine and topical epinephrine (1:10000) for over 10 minutes. The bleeding region can then be cauterised using a silver nitrate stick.

   e **True.** Shock is an important and lethal complication, especially in elderly patients.

2. a **True.** Intermittent bouts of sneezing are a common feature of allergic rhinitis.

   b **False.** Patients with allergic rhinitis tend to have a clear discharge (rhinorrhoea) rather than a bloody one (epistaxis).

c **True.** Rhinorrhoea refers to a discharge from the nose. It occurs in colds and upper respiratory tract infections, but also in allergic rhinitis.

d **False.** Patients with allergic rhinitis tend to sneeze rather than cough.

e **True.** Due to the inflammatory response occurring within the nose, the mucosal linings swell. This may result in a patient complaining of a blocked nose in allergic rhinitis.

3. a **True.** This may be either topical or systemic antihistamine medication. Unfortunately, traditional antihistamines cross the blood–brain barrier, resulting in drowsiness. Modern antihistamines do not cross the blood–brain barrier, and so do not cause this unwanted side-effect.

b **True.** These are effective for the symptomatic relief of allergic rhinitis.

c **True.** This is an important intervention. It may involve removing pets, changing diet or changing mattresses/pillows. The allergen that is causing allergic rhinitis must first be identified, and then appropriate avoidance practices can be put in place.

d **False.** Since allergic rhinitis is an immune condition resulting from stimulation of receptors on the nasal mucosal lining, ligating the olfactory nerve will have no effect on this condition other than irreversibly removing the sense of smell. Turbinate resection can help congestive symptoms, although this procedure is reserved for severe cases which have not responded to medical therapy.

e **True.** This is a relatively new therapy, and it is not as widely available as other possible treatments. For this reason it is reserved for those patients who have more severe symptoms. It involves exposing the patient to the allergen in minute doses which do not trigger an allergic reaction, and slowly increasing this dose over time. Because of the hazardous nature of this therapy and the risk of anaphylaxis, it must be undertaken in hospital or at a location that has sufficient expertise and equipment to provide resuscitation if necessary.

4. a **True.** Symptoms that are exacerbated by pollen and other plant material are classed as hayfever or seasonal allergic rhinitis, as this condition is most common in the summer months.

b **True.**

c **True.**

d **False.** Plastic is not a common cause of allergic rhinitis.

e **True.**

5. a **False.** Allergic rhinitis is an immune-mediated condition, whereas intrinsic rhinitis is a neuronally mediated condition. Medical treatment is similar for the two conditions, although allergen avoidance will not benefit a patient who has intrinsic allergic rhinitis.

b **True.** Rhinitis medicamentosa is the name given to the rebound nasal congestion that occurs after using nasal decongestant agents continuously for over a week. Continuous use of nasal decongestants can result in nasal obstruction secondary to turbinate hyperplasia.

c **True.** Allergic rhinitis is a type 1 hypersensitivity reaction.

d **False.** Allergic rhinitis is IgE mediated, as are all type 1 hypersensitivity reactions.

e **False.** Atopic conditions include allergies, eczema and asthma. Patients with allergic rhinitis are more likely to suffer from any of these conditions.

6. a **True.** Nasal polyps can independently increase congestion and thus predispose to infection.

b **True.** This is a common presentation.

c **False.** Nasal polyps are present in the nose. They cannot cause a neck lump.

d **False.** There is no link between nasal polyps and salivation.

e **True.** Nasal polyps are sacs of oedematous mucosa and they can cause rhinorrhoea.

7. a **True.** Continuous infection and subsequent inflammation predispose to polyp formation.

b **True.**

c **True.**

d **False.**

e **True.**

8. a **False.** This will quickly result in rhinitis medicamentosa, in which rebound swelling of the nasal mucosa will occur.

b **False.** This is too extreme for nasal polyps. Radiotherapy is not used in the treatment of nasal polyps.

c **False.** Nasal polyps do not contain the rapidly dividing cancerous cells that are targeted by chemotherapy. Unlike polyps in the large bowel, nasal polyps are not cancerous, and chemotherapy has no role in their treatment.

d **True.** This is a useful option for helping to decrease the size of the polyps.

e **True.** The polyps can be removed through the nostrils.

9. a **False.** If several attempts to remove the foreign body have failed, the patient should be given a general anaesthetic and a further attempt made in theatre. Repeated unsuccessful attempts to remove a foreign object merely increase the trauma to the surrounding tissues.

b **False.** Inorganic material does not decay. Both organic and inorganic foreign bodies should be removed due to the risk of inhalation.

c **True.** A foul-smelling discharge may accompany an organic foreign body that has been in place for an extended period of time.

d **False.** They are more common in children.

e **False.** There is no ethnic variation in the incidence.

10. a **True.** The common cold is a common cause of rhinorrhoea. The discharge is usually clear and may be caused by rhinovirus or adenovirus. There are a number of other upper respiratory tract viruses that may also be causal agents.

b **False.** *E. coli* is not a virus, nor does it cause the common cold. It is implicated in gastrointestinal symptoms.

c **True.**

d **False.** Epstein–Barr virus does not cause the common cold. It is responsible for infectious mononucleosis.

e **False.** This virus has been implicated in cervical cancer and laryngeal cancer, but does not have a role in the aetiology of the common cold.

11. a **True.** Rhinorrhoea is the term used to describe nasal discharge. It aids the spread (in droplet and aerosol form) of the viruses that cause the common cold.

b **False.** The common cold is an upper respiratory tract infection and does not cause diarrhoea.

c **True.** Sneezing also occurs in the common cold, and is an effective method of spreading the viruses that cause this condition between hosts.

d **False.** The common cold does not cause haematemesis.

e **True.** This is due to the nasal membranes swelling and becoming engorged.

12. a **True.** Topical decongestants used modestly can provide symptomatic relief of the congestive symptoms of the common cold.
   b **True.** Steam inhalation is a difficult technique to perform correctly, but it does help to clear the nasal passages and provide some relief of congestive symptoms.
   c **False.** Rest and conservative measures are the most effective way to recover from the common cold.
   d **True.** Paracetamol is an excellent choice of medication for the common cold, due to its antipyrexial and analgesic properties.
   e **False.** The common cold is caused by viruses, not bacteria. Therefore antibiotics will not be of any use for treating it.

13. a **True.** Periorbital cellulitis is a serious complication of ethmoidal sinusitis.
   b **True.** Frontal lobe sinusitis can give rise to frontal lobe abscesses. This can present as a sudden change in personality or as strange behaviour.
   c **True.** Frontal lobe sinusitis can give rise to extradural, subdural and frontal lobe abscesses, meningitis and osteomyelitis.
   d **False.** Rhinorrhoea or nasal discharge is a normal symptom in sinusitis and, in the absence of confusion and other signs, does not indicate a serious complication.
   e **True.** Cavernous sinus thrombosis can give rise to ophthalmoplegia and proptosis.

14. a **True.** Syphilis can cause septal perforation.
   b **False.** SLE does not affect the nose.
   c **True.** Wegener's granulomatosis is a granulomatous disease that can affect the nose.
   d **False.** Osteoarthritis is a degenerative disease that does not affect the nose.
   e **True.** Sarcoidosis can cause nasal granulomas.

15. a **True.** Cocaine causes vasoconstriction of nasal arterioles, which can in turn result in ischaemic nasal perforation.
   b **True.** Nasal trauma can result in an acute septal perforation. Chronic trauma, such as nose picking, can also result in perforation in extreme cases.
   c **False.** Sneezing does not result in nasal septal perforation.

  d **False.** Heroin, unlike cocaine, does not cause septal perforation.

  e **True.** Syphilis is a granulomatous disease, and can result in septal perforation.

16. a **False.** There is no relationship between vocal cord polyps and nasal septal deviation.

  b **True.**

  c **False.**

  d **False.**

  e **True.** A broken nose commonly results in septal deviation.

17. a **True.** Visibly they appear similar to nasal polyps.

  b **False.** They arise from the maxillary sinus.

  c **False.** Nasal polyps are commonly found bilaterally. Antrochoanal polyps usually arise unilaterally in the nasopharynx, not from within the nostril itself.

  d **False.** Nasal polyps may respond to nasal topical steroids. However, antrochoanal polyps require surgery.

  e **True.** Antrochoanal polyps require surgical intervention.

18. a **True.** Periorbital cellulitis may be a serious complication of ethmoidal sinusitis.

  b **True.** This is a serious condition, and a multi-disciplinary approach should be sought.

  c **True.** Upper respiratory tract infection can lead to sinusitis. Periorbital cellulitis can result from ethmoidal sinusitis.

  d **True.** This is a serious condition and it requires intravenous broad-spectrum antibiotics.

  e **True.** This is due to infection of the tissues around the eye.

19. a **True.** A thorough history should explain the mechanism of any trauma.

  b **True.** Even though dental matters are beyond the remit of medical practitioners, there is no reason why you cannot make a brief inspection of dental hygiene. Dental decay can give rise to cheek swelling and pain. Palpating the relevant tooth will elicit this pain.

  c **True.** Be sure to take a full occupational and social history. Sinus cancer can often have subtle signs. Ask about rhinitis and epistaxis.

  d **False.** This is just another name for a pharyngeal pouch. This is found in the pharynx and commonly presents with dysphagia.

It is not one of the first diagnoses to consider when a patient presents with a cheek swelling.

e **False.** Tympanic membrane perforation describes perforation of the eardrum. It usually occurs secondary to a build-up of pressure due to external trauma, middle ear effusion or infection.

20. a **False.** Nasal manipulation is usually performed 10–14 days after the injury, as this is the ideal time for stable reduction.

b **True.** In fact there is a good chance that the procedure will not produce a perfect cosmetic result. The patient must be made aware of this, to avoid disappointment with the result. In view of this, it is very important to have a photographic record of what the patient looked like before and after the procedure. He should be made aware of the cosmetic surgical options at a later date if he so wishes.

c **False.** This procedure will attempt to straighten the nose. It will not treat any internal septal deviation. The patient may require a further procedure to deal with this if it causes him problems.

d **True.** He may require an external splint if the manipulated nasal position is likely to deviate. The nasal position can be held in place by the splint for several days after the procedure.

e **True.** He should be warned that the procedure may cause bleeding, but he should be reassured that it will be managed effectively in theatre.

21. a **True.**

b **False.** The patient does not have any greater incidence of lower respiratory tract infection.

c **True.** Bleeding can be a problem if the patient has any bleeding disorders or is on any antiplatelet or anticoagulant medication. A thorough history will help to elucidate this.

d **True.**

e **True.** This is transient and soon disappears.

22. a **True.** This is an unfortunate complication of this procedure, and may result in a whistling sound on breathing, as well as nasal dryness.

b **True.** The patient should be advised what to look for after a septoplasty. A septal haematoma can cause irreparable cartilage necrosis, and presents with nasal blockage and pain. It requires urgent drainage.

c **True.** This is especially true if the patient is suffering from accompanying rhinitis. The rhinitis may continue to cause nasal obstruction despite the fact that the septal deviation has been treated.

d **True.** The patient may feel nasal blockage for a long time after the procedure, but he should be reassured that the symptoms will diminish with time.

e **True.** The patient should not be alarmed by this, but if bleeding continues for an extended period of time he should be advised to return to the hospital.

23. a **True.** The triad of Wegener's granulomatosis includes glomerulonephritis, respiratory tract granulomas and vasculitis.

b **False.** Bowel cancer is not directly associated with Wegener's granulomatosis.

c **True.** Epistaxis and rhinorrhoea are the early signs of Wegener's granulomatosis. They provide a prompt to ask further questions in order to ascertain whether any other organ systems have been affected. It is important to keep rare conditions such as this in mind, and not to overlook them when assessing patients. Cytoplasmic pattern anti-neutrophil cytoplasmic antibody (c-ANCA) is a very specific test to confirm the diagnosis.

d **False.** Osteoporosis is not directly associated with Wegener's granulomatosis.

e **True.** Immunosuppression is the mainstay of treatment for this condition. Agents such as methotrexate, azathioprine and steroids are used to control symptoms.

24. a **False.** These tumours occur in the region of the cheek. There is no relationship between such tumours and a change in bowel habit.

b **False.** Maxillary antrum cancer does not cause heart palpitations.

c **True.** Nasal obstruction is often bilateral, so the nature of unilateral nasal obstruction should be explored in greater detail.

d **False.** Maxillary antrum cancer does not cause back pain.

e **True.** Patients may complain of a bloody nasal discharge. They may also complain of pain with a visible swelling over the maxillary region. You must always conduct a careful lymphatic examination in any patient whom you suspect has a head and neck cancer.

25. a **True.** Trauma is the usual cause of a septal haematoma.

b **True.** The patient's temperature should be carefully taken in order to rule out fever due to infection. The formation of a septal abscess can be avoided by timely drainage of the haematoma.

c **False.** It may result in ischaemia and perforation of the septal cartilage.

d **True.** The saddle-nose deformity may result from an untreated septal haematoma. It will require cosmetic surgery to correct it, and could easily have been avoided by early treatment of the haematoma.

e **True.** Large haematomas may need to be drained.

26. a **True.** The subsequent nasal congestion from nasal polyps results in anosmia.

b **False.** Middle ear infection does not directly cause anosmia.

c **True.** Nasal drug use can result in anosmia. Cocaine in particular causes vasoconstriction and ischaemia, with subsequent anosmia.

d **False.** Cancer of the salivary glands has no direct impact on the sense of smell.

e **True.** These prevent sensory perception from reaching the brain, and thus result in anosmia.

27. a **False.** Rhinorrhoea is rarely unilateral and incidentally post-traumatic. The history of trauma suggests that the discharge could be cerebrospinal fluid.

b **False.** Nasal polyps tend to be bilateral and cause nasal obstruction. It is very unlikely that the clinical picture and sudden onset of symptoms are due to a nasal polyp.

c **False.** The pterion is situated on the lateral aspect of the skull. It is an anatomical weak point, and the middle meningeal artery runs deeps to it. Trauma to this part of the head will result in an epidural haematoma. The clinical picture in this case does not correlate with such an injury. The watery cerebrospinal fluid leak and anosmia are better explained by a fracture of the anterior fossa or cribriform plate.

d **True.** There has been a fracture, and the transparent watery nasal discharge is in fact cerebrospinal fluid (CSF).

e **True.** This is the most likely source of the CSF leak, as it explains the patient's accompanying anosmia.

28. a **True.** This causes the minority of cases of acute bacterial sinusitis. It is an aerobic Gram-negative diplococcal bacterium that can colonise the respiratory tract. Up to 5% of colds can progress to acute bacterial sinusitis. It is important to have a basic idea of the likely pathogens, as treatment is with antibiotics.

b **False.** As suggested by its name, adenovirus is a virus, not a bacterium. It can cause the common cold. Acute bacterial sinusitis is caused by bacterial infection secondary to a viral infection.

c **True.** This is the most common cause of acute bacterial sinusitis. It is a Gram-positive, alpha-haemolytic bacterium that is generally an anaerobe.

d **False.** *E. coli* is a Gram-negative facultative anaerobe that is commonly found in the lower gastrointestinal tract. It does not cause acute bacterial sinusitis.

e **True.** *Haemophilus influenzae* is a Gram-negative facultative anaerobe, and may cause up to a third of cases of acute bacterial sinusitis.

29. a **True.** This is a difficult question, but the triad of conditions that make up chronic inflammatory sinusitis include nasal polyps, asthma and NSAID sensitivity (especially to aspirin). This is also known as Samter's triad.

b **False.** This is not part of the triad of symptoms that make up chronic inflammatory sinusitis.

c **True.** This is particularly true of aspirin.

d **True.** Bronchial asthma is also part of the triad. You should be wary about prescribing NSAIDs to any asthmatic patient, not just those diagnosed with chronic inflammatory sinusitis.

e **False.** This is not part of the triad of symptoms that make up chronic inflammatory sinusitis.

30. a **True.** This question requires you to combine and apply your knowledge of two separate conditions. Patients with cystic fibrosis have thick mucus secretions due to abnormal exchange of chloride ions. Cystic fibrosis is an autosomal recessive disorder caused by a mutation at the CFTR gene on the long arm of chromosome 7.

b **False.** There is no link between HIV and cystic fibrosis.

c **True.** Patients with cystic fibrosis have a higher incidence of nasal polyps. These can exacerbate congestion and thus sinusitis.

d **True.** It is often difficult to eradicate any infection, due to the viscosity of the mucus in the sinuses. Mucolytic agents help to loosen the mucus and thus assist in its removal.

e **True.**

31. a **True.** This question assesses whether the candidate can appreciate the differences in sinusitis among different patient groups.

HIV is an immunocompromised state, and this is reflected by the range of pathogens that can be isolated from the sinuses of patients with this condition.

b **True.**

c **False.** This is associated with laryngeal cancer, but has no direct aetiological link with sinusitis in HIV patients.

d **False.** Epstein–Barr virus is associated with nasopharyngeal cancer, but has no direct aetiological link with sinusitis in HIV patients.

e **True.**

32. a **True.** There are many viruses that can cause rhinitis. Others include parainfluenza virus and enterovirus.

 b **False.** *Staphylococcus aureus* is a bacterium and does not cause rhinitis. Always read the question carefully. This one is asking for viruses, not bacteria.

 c **False.** *Haemophilus influenzae* is not a virus and does not cause rhinitis.

 d **False.** This virus is responsible for cervical cancer and laryngeal cancer. It does not directly cause rhinitis.

 e **True.** Rhinovirus is commonly associated with the common cold and rhinitis.

33. a **True.** Nasal polyps can cause nasal discharge.

 b **False.** There is no link between a urinary tract infection and rhinitis.

 c **True.** Allergy is a common cause of rhinitis.

 d **True.** Vasomotor rhinitis results from dilation of blood vessels causing increased mucus production.

 e **True.** The viruses that are responsible for the common cold commonly cause rhinitis.

34. a **True.** By week 4, the neural crest cells migrate towards the middle of the face and mark the foundation of the development of the nose.

 b **True.** The development of the nose ultimately begins during week 4 of gestation.

 c **False.** The nose begins to develop by week 4 of gestation.

 d **False.** The nasal conchi form much later, during weeks 25–28 of gestation.

 e **True.** These placodes ultimately help to form the nasal cavity.

35. a **True.** The facial pain associated with acute sinusitis may be worse on coughing or leaning forward.

b **False.** Vomiting is not a feature of acute sinusitis.

c **True.** The maxillary sinus is commonly affected in acute sinusitis, and can present with pain in this region.

d **True.** Nasal obstruction occurs when the swollen nasal mucosa in acute sinusitis prevents normal air entry.

e **True.** When taking a history from a patient who is complaining of facial pain, nasal obstruction and congestion, particular care should be taken to establish the chronological sequence of events. In acute sinusitis, an upper respiratory tract infection usually precedes the onset of these symptoms.

36. a **True.** This surgical technique uses diathermy to burn the submucosal tissue and thereby reduce the swelling produced by turbinate hypertrophy. At the other extreme, cryotherapy can also be used to destroy mucosal tissue by freezing it.

b **False.** Turbinate hypertrophy is usually secondary to allergic rhinitis. As a result, a tonsillectomy plays no role in reducing the size of the turbinates, nor do the tonsils have a role in the aetiology of turbinate hypertrophy.

c **False.** Myringectomy is a surgical procedure that involves perforation of the tympanic membrane. This procedure has no role in the treatment of turbinate hypertrophy.

d **True.** This technique removes a part of the turbinate, thereby reducing nasal cavity obstruction.

e **False.** Perforating the nasal septum will not help to reduce turbinate hypertrophy.

37. a **True.** Unilateral nasal discharge is an important sign when considering the possibility of a retained nasal foreign body.

b **True.** A retained foreign body results in infection. If it is not removed, chronic infection can be manifested as sinusitis, and antibiotics will be of little use unless the foreign body is removed.

c **True.** The foreign body will create an obstruction and thus cause difficulty in nasal breathing.

d **False.** There is no association between a retained nasal foreign body and cataract formation.

e **False.** Chvostek's sign is elicited by tapping over the cheek on the side of the face. Facial twitching in response to this action is suggestive of hypocalcaemia, which can be a complication of thyroid surgery (due to unintended damage to the parathyroid glands) or a result of parathyroid gland pathology. Chvostek's sign is not elicited in patients with a retained nasal foreign body.

38. a **True.** Acute nasal deformity is usually a result of direct trauma. This is an indication to examine within the nose for septal haematoma formation. Septal haematomas occur between the nasal septum and perichondrium layer.
    b **True.** The swelling may distort the septum, causing an asymmetrical appearance.
    c **False.** It usually takes between 1 and 3 days for a septal haematoma to form. It does not form immediately after injury.
    d **True.** The septal haematoma may be palpated by the examiner. Care should be taken to ensure that gloves are worn during the examination.
    e **False.** A septal haematoma should be drained as soon as possible in order to prevent ischaemic necrosis of the nasal cartilage.

39. a **True.** The septal haematoma can cause the nose structure to collapse and result in a saddle-nose deformity.
    b **True.** Septal perforation can occur due to ischaemic necrosis of the nasal cartilage if the septal haematoma is not drained quickly.
    c **False.** Dysphagia refers to difficulty in swallowing, and is not a feature of a septal haematoma.
    d **True.** The haematoma can become infected, resulting in septal abscess formation. This can lead to the development of systemic symptoms such as fever and malaise.
    e **False.** Ventricular fibrillation is a life-threatening heart arrhythmia, and is not caused by a septal haematoma.

40. a **False.** There is no association between laryngeal cancer and sinusitis.
    b **True.** This is a serious complication that must be suspected in all patients with sinusitis and erythematous swollen skin around the eye.
    c **False.** Dysuria refers to pain during urination. It is not a feature of sinusitis.
    d **False.** Otosclerosis involves the gradual fixation of the ossicles due to bone changes. It is not related to sinusitis.
    e **True.** This is a serious complication that requires urgent intravenous antibiotics. It may present with personality change, and may require surgery to evacuate the abscess.

41. a **False.** Epiphora is the term used to describe excessive tear production. It is due to the inability of the tears to drain naturally through the superior and inferior canaliculi down via the lacrimal sac into the nasolacrimal duct and then to enter the nasal cavity.

  b **False.** In epiphora the eyes are excessively watery due to the fact that the tears cannot drain away. Therefore these patients will not benefit from eye drops.

  c **True.** As explained above, the eyes are excessively watery due to a problem with the drainage of tears into the nasal cavity.

  d **False.** Epiphora has a good prognosis when treated using endoscopic dacryocystorhinostomy (DCR).

  e **True.** Endoscopic DCR is a surgical procedure that involves inserting a tiny drainage tube to connect the superior and inferior canaliculi to the nasolacrimal duct. This allows tear drainage and alleviates the patient's symptoms. It is successful in the vast majority of cases. The use of an endoscopic approach reduces the length of the patient's hospital stay, as well as the likelihood of complications and the invasiveness of the procedure.

42. a **False.** Endoscopic DCR involves making a small connection between the lacrimal sac and the nasal cavity. There are no external incisions or subsequent scars.

  b **False.** The whole point of endoscopic DCR is to avoid external incisions and thus facial scars. Any scarring occurs internally and is not visible.

  c **False.** Endoscopic DCR is a quick and minimally invasive procedure that can be performed as a simple day case.

  d **True.** One of the advantages of an endoscopic technique is that the length of hospital stay is reduced due to the minimally invasive nature of the procedure. Endoscopic DCR is a relatively quick procedure, and the patient can leave hospital the same day.

  e **False.** Endoscopic DCR can be performed under general or local anaesthetic, but cannot be performed under spinal block anaesthesia.

43. a **True.** Part of the nose around the site of intervention can feel congested due to the natural inflammatory response to surgery. This is normal, and will resolve spontaneously within 1 week after surgery.

  b **True.** Although it is usually negligible, bleeding is a possible complication of endoscopic DCR surgery.

    c **False.** Coughing is not a complication of endoscopic DCR surgery.

    d **False.** Anosmia refers to loss of the sense of smell. It is not a complication of endoscopic DCR surgery.

    e **True.** The drainage devices can be well concealed and consequently difficult to remove 3 months after the procedure.

44. a **True.** The drainage of the maxillary sinus opens into the hiatus semilunaris in the middle meatus just inferior to the middle concha.

    b **True.** The frontonasal duct opens into the hiatus semilunaris inferior to the middle concha, and is responsible for draining the anterior ethmoidal and frontal sinus. The middle aspect of the ethmoid sinus also flows into the middle meatus via the bulla ethmoidalis, but the posterior aspect of the ethmoid sinus drains into the superior meatus.

    c **False.** The sphenoethmoidal sinus drains into the sphenoethmoidal recess between the roof of the nasal cavity and the superior concha.

    d **False.** The nasolacrimal duct opens into the inferior meatus just beneath the inferior concha.

    e **False.** The posterior ethmoid sinus actually drains into the superior meatus under the superior concha. Both the anterior and middle ethmoid sinuses drain into the middle meatus. The anterior aspect of the ethmoid sinus drains into the hiatus semilunaris via the frontonasal duct, and the middle aspect of the ethmoid sinus drains out of the bulla ethmoidalis.

45. a **False.** The conchae are mucosa-lined bony protrusions from the lateral aspect of the nasal cavity. The most important function of the conchae is to help to humidify and warm the nasally inspired air. There are three conchae in each nasal cavity, and thus a total of six overall for the whole nose. These are the superior, middle and inferior conchae (named after their anatomical locations). The superior and middle conchae arise from the ethmoidal bone, and the inferior concha arises from the maxillary bone.

    b **False.** The conchae protrude from the lateral wall of the nasal cavity.

    c **False.** The meatus is the name given to the space between the shelves of conchae through which nasally inspired and expired air travels. There are three conchae, on each side, and three correspondingly named meatuses. For instance, the space between the inferior concha and the nasal floor is called the inferior meatus, and the space between the inferior and middle conchae is called the middle meatus. The space between the middle and superior conchae is called the superior meatus. The space between the superior meatus and the nasal roof is called the sphenoethmoidal recess.

d **False.** The conchae help to warm the inspired air.

e **False.** The conchae help to humidify the inspired air.

46. a **False.** The sense of smell is mediated by the olfactory nerve, which is the first of the cranial nerves. The oculomotor nerve is responsible for various movements of the eye, in addition to the autonomic innervation of the eye.

b **False.** Anosmia is the term used to describe complete loss of the sense of smell.

c **False.** The facial nerve supplies the muscles of facial expression and sensation to the anterior two-thirds of the tongue. It also innervates the submandibular and sublingual glands. In addition, it inner-vates an anatomically variable region around the external acoustic meatus. The olfactory nerve is responsible for the sense of smell.

d **True.** Infective or inflammatory conditions can result in swell-ing of the nasal mucosa and the production of nasal discharge. Cumulatively these can physically prevent odour molecules from stimulating the olfactory nerve in the roof of the nasal cavity.

e **True.** Smell is mediated via cyclic AMP and a G-protein cascade mechanism.

47. a **False.** The superficial layer consists of pseudostratified columnar epithelium in addition to goblet cells. These cells sit on a base-ment membrane overlying the lamina propria layer.

b **True.** Goblet cells secrete the mucous lining of the nasal mucosa.

c **True.** The superficial layer of the nasal mucosa consists of columnar cells that have tiny hair-like projections (cilia that aid the movement of the overlying mucus).

d **False.** Astrocytes are a type of neuronal glial cell found within the nervous system. They do not occur within the nasal mucosa.

e **True.** This layer contains a vast network of small blood vessels that feed the rich supply of mucus-secreting cells in the nasal mucosa, and thus warm and humidify the inflowing air.

48. a **True.** The external nasal branch of the ophthalmic division of the trigeminal nerve innervates the anterior aspect of the nose,

whereas the infraorbital branch of the maxillary division of the trigeminal nerve innervates the lateral aspect of the nose.

b **False.** The cochlear nerve is responsible for hearing. It does not innervate the nasal septum.

c **False.** The optic nerve is responsible for vision. The olfactory nerve innervates the sense of smell. However, caustic odours are sensed by the trigeminal nerve.

d **True.** The olfactory nerve axons descend through the perforations in the cribriform plate to detect odours.

e **True.** The ethmoid bone gives rise to the cribriform plate through which the olfactory nerve axons descend.

49. a **True.** Von Willebrand disease is caused by a deficiency in von Willebrand factor, and is the commonest inherited coagulation problem. Bleeding is difficult to control in these patients, as without von Willebrand factor the platelets have difficulty adhering to each other.

b **True.** Warfarin is an anticoagulant that prevents blood clot formation. Therefore bleeding in these patients will be more difficult to control.

c **True.** Vitamin K is important for various clotting factors, and its deficiency results in prolonged bleeding.

d **False.** Thalassaemia is a genetic condition in which patients have abnormal haemoglobin and can suffer from anaemia.

e **True.** Haemophilia is an inherited condition in which bleeding is prolonged due to impaired coagulation.

50. a **False.** Rhinoplasty is the term used to describe reconstruction of the nose, whereas septoplasty refers to reconstruction of the nasal septum.

b **True.** Rhinoplasty can be performed for functional reasons, such as reconstructing the nose to improve airflow in particular patients.

c **False.** Rhinoplasty refers to reconstruction of the nose.

d **True.** Periorbital bruising tends to recover soon after the procedure. However, there may be facial and nasal swelling which can take longer to resolve as the tissue heals.

e **True.** Rhinoplasty can be performed for cosmetic reasons.

51. a **False.** The superior meatus is located between the superior and middle conchae. The sphenoethmoidal recess is located between the nasal roof and the superior concha.

b **False.** The frontal sinus drains via the frontonasal duct into the middle meatus by an opening in the hiatus semilunaris.

c **True.** The nasolacrimal duct opens just beneath the inferior concha into the inferior meatus.

d **False.** The inferior meatus is located between the floor of the nasal cavity and the inferior concha. The middle meatus is located between the middle and inferior conchae.

e **False.** Tears from the lacrimal sac are drained via the nasolacrimal duct into the inferior meatus. This is why a runny nose often accompanies crying.

52. a **True.** This Gram-positive coccus is commonly found in the nose.

b **False.** *E. coli* is a Gram-negative bacterium found in the lower gastrointestinal tract. It is not part of the normal nasal flora.

c **True.** This Gram-positive coccus is commonly found in the nose.

d **True.** This is a Gram-negative rod that can be found in the nasal flora.

e **False.** This Gram-negative bacterium can cause gastric ulcers. It is not found as part of the normal nasal mucosa.

53. a **True.** This is a Gram-negative rod that can be found in the nasal flora.

b **False.** This Gram-negative intracellular organism is responsible for a sexually transmitted infection and is not found in the nasal flora.

c **False.** This Gram-positive coccus is non-pathogenic.

d **False.** *Legionella pneumophila* is a Gram-negative bacterium that is the cause of the pneumonia in Legionnaires' disease.

e **True.** It is a Gram-positive, alpha-haemolytic bacterium that is generally an anaerobe. It can prove pathogenic in certain circumstances, and can infect many different tissues.

54. a **False.** The sphenoid sinus is not as well developed in children as it is in adults. The maxillary sinus is usually most commonly affected in children.

b **True.** Sinusitis, like many other infections, causes the body to respond with a fever.

c **False.** *Helicobacter pylori* is a bacterium that attacks the gastric mucosa and causes gastric ulcers. *Staphylococcus aureus* and streptococci are common causes of sinusitis in children.

d **True.** Bacterial sinusitis in children will respond to antibiotics.

e **False.** The presentation of sinusitis in children is very similar to that in adults. Nasal congestion and rhinorrhoea are common. However, vomiting is not seen in sinusitis.

55. a **True.** The narrowest part of the nasal passage is at the front, between the septum and the inferior turbinates. This area is known as the nasal valve.

b **True.** The cause of septal deviation in a patient is often unknown.

c **True.** There is a natural cycle of engorgement of the tissues of the nose from one side to the other every 8 hours. This engorgement is exaggerated in hayfever (seasonal rhinitis), hence the nasal obstruction.

d **True.** Neonates are obligate (compulsory) nasal breathers. For this reason a congenital obstruction of the posterior choani (openings at the back of the nose) can lead to asphyxia unless corrective measures are taken.

e **True.**

The throat

Questions

1. The following are causes of a chronic cough:
   a Gastro-oesophageal reflux disease (GORD).
   b Angiotensin-converting-enzyme (ACE) inhibitor medication.
   c Asthma.
   d Post-nasal drip.
   e Smoking.

2. Regarding glottic stenosis, the following statements are true:
   a It may be congenital in origin.
   b It refers to narrowing at the level of the tonsils.
   c It may result from intubation for longer than 2 weeks.
   d It may present with dysphonia.
   e It may present with epistaxis.

3. Regarding vocal cord nodules, the following statements are true:
   a They are more common in singers.
   b They may present with a hoarse voice.
   c They should be surgically removed immediately, regardless of the severity of the symptoms.
   d The patient should be advised that the more they strain their voice, the faster recovery will be.
   e They are an autosomal dominant condition.

4. Risk factors for laryngeal cancer include the following:
   a Excess chronic alcohol consumption.
   b Age less than 20 years.
   c Eating spicy food.
   d Smoking.
   e Male gender.

5. Laryngeal cancer may present with the following symptoms:
   a Dysphagia.
   b Weight gain.
   c Malaise.
   d Neck swelling.
   e Bloody sputum.

6. Indications for a tonsillectomy include the following:
   a Chronic tonsillitis.
   b Presence of a bleeding disorder.
   c Obstructive sleep apnoea.
   d A BMI of 35 kg/m².
   e Recurrent tonsillitis.

7. Regarding stridor, the following statements are true:
   a Stridor is synonymous with stertor.
   b Stridor is an abnormal breathing sound that is heard in inspiration, and which is caused by a narrowed airway above the level of the larynx.
   c Stridor is an abnormal breathing sound that is caused by a narrowed airway below the level of the larynx.
   d Stridor is always inspiratory when present.
   e Stridor may originate from narrowing of the bronchioles.

8. The following are causes of stridor:
   a Asthma.
   b Epiglottitis.
   c Croup.
   d Adenoid hypertrophy.
   e Laryngeal cancer.

9. The following are causes of stertor:
   a Tonsillar hypertrophy.
   b Chronic obstructive pulmonary disease (COPD).
   c Adenoid hypertrophy.
   d Nasal obstruction.
   e Acute laryngitis.

10. Regarding epiglottitis, the following statements are true:
    a It is caused by *Haemophilus influenzae* group B.
    b Diagnosis must be made by inspecting the back of the throat, regardless of any distress this may cause the child.
    c It may present with temperature, stridor and dribbling.
    d Vaccination may prevent this disease.
    e Epiglottitis is a medical emergency.

11. Regarding croup, the following statements are true:
    a It is also known as laryngotracheobronchitis.
    b It may be caused by parainfluenza virus.
    c Treatment may involve nebulised steroids and beta-receptor agonists.
    d It is most common in teenagers.
    e It commonly requires a tracheostomy.

12. The following may be causes of chronic dysphagia:
    a Myasthenia gravis.
    b Multiple sclerosis.
    c Vocal cord nodule.
    d Thyroid cancer.
    e Globus pharyngeus.

13. Regarding dysphonia, the following statements are true:
    a It describes complete loss of voice.
    b If the dysphonia lasts for more than 4 weeks, an urgent ENT referral is indicated.
    c It may be caused by bronchial carcinoma.
    d It is improved by smoking.
    e It may be due to a vocal cord polyp.

14. The following are complications of tracheostomy:
    a Otalgia.
    b Infection.
    c Surgical emphysema.
    d Haemorrhage.
    e Tube blockage.

15. Causes of chronic pharyngitis include the following:
   a Gastro-oesophageal reflux disease (GORD).
   b Smoking.
   c Alcohol.
   d Vitamin D deficiency.
   e Heart failure.

16. With regard to swallowing, the following statements are true:
   a The swallowing process consists of the oral, pharyngeal and oesophageal phases.
   b All of the phases of the swallowing process are under involuntary control.
   c The vagus and glossopharyngeal nerves are involved in the swallowing reflex.
   d Bulbar palsy causes difficulty in the swallowing movement.
   e Achalasia causes difficulty in swallowing.

17. Voice abusers are at risk of the following conditions:
   a Reinke's oedema.
   b Epiglottitis.
   c Vocal nodules.
   d Tonsillitis.
   e Capillary ectasia.

18. The following anatomy is involved in speaking:
   a The vocal cords.
   b The tongue.
   c The teeth.
   d The lips.
   e The lungs.

19. Regarding endotracheal intubation, the following statements are true:
   a It is slower and more dangerous to perform than tracheostomy.
   b In children, a tracheostomy is safer than endotracheal intubation.
   c Endotracheal intubation expertise is more readily available than tracheostomy expertise.
   d Endotracheal intubation may be used as a safe airway for several months before changing.
   e If placed incorrectly, it may result in ventilation entering the stomach.

20. The following statements are true of enlarged adenoids:
    a Sleep apnoea may be present.
    b Glue ear may be present.
    c Dysphagia may be present.
    d Nasal discharge and nasal speech may be present.
    e They are more common in the elderly.

21. Regarding pharyngeal pouch, the following statements are true:
    a It may present with dysphagia.
    b It may be palpable as a swelling in the neck.
    c It is a common inherited disease affecting 1 in 100 people.
    d Barium swallow may demonstrate the pharyngeal pouch.
    e It can be treated endoscopically.

22. Regarding angioedema of the larynx, the following statements are true:
    a It is a medical emergency.
    b It requires an intramuscular injection of adrenaline.
    c The patient should be sent home as soon as the swelling has disappeared.
    d It may be caused by an allergy.
    e It requires immediate tracheostomy.

23. The following are investigations used to diagnose pathologies of the larynx and pharynx:
    a Fibre-optic nasendoscopy.
    b Barium swallow.
    c Lumbar puncture.
    d CT scan.
    e D-dimer test.

24. The following symptoms may be present if a foreign body has been swallowed:
    a Pooling of saliva.
    b Epistaxis.
    c Pain in the neck.
    d Otalgia.
    e Coughing.

25. The following symptoms may be present if a foreign body has been inhaled:
    a Wheezing.
    b Choking.
    c Tinnitus.
    d Dyspnoea.
    e Coughing.

26. A 32-year-old man, while laughing at the dinner table during his meal, begins to choke and is starting to turn blue. Fortunately you are present at a nearby table. The following statements are true regarding the initial management of this patient:
    a The patient has swallowed a foreign body.
    b The Heimlich manoeuvre should be attempted.
    c The Heimlich manoeuvre involves giving two breaths and 30 chest compressions.
    d Obstruction of the right bronchus is more dangerous than obstruction of the larynx.
    e The patient will recover spontaneously and should not be approached.

27. Regarding laryngeal papillomatosis, the following statements are true:
    a It is caused by human papillomavirus.
    b It may present with stridor or hoarseness.
    c It should be left untreated as it is self-limiting.
    d It may cause complete airway obstruction.
    e It is usually acquired from the mother.

28. Regarding globus pharyngeus, the following statements are true:
    a It is the sensation of a lump in the ear.
    b It requires a pharyngectomy.
    c It is a premalignant condition.
    d It is more common in patients with psychological conditions.
    e It can be investigated using an ECG.

29. The following predispose to obstructive sleep apnoea:
    a Smoking.
    b Obesity.
    c Drinking tea.
    d Alcohol.
    e Large tonsils and adenoids.

30. A mother brings a 9-year-old child to see you regarding his recurrent tonsillitis. She claims that he has had eight episodes during the last year and seven episodes the previous year. This has resulted in a lot of time away from school, and he frequently complains of a sore throat. Which of the features in the history suggest that a tonsillectomy may be appropriate?
    a He has had more than one attack in the last year.
    b Symptoms have persisted for more than 1 year.
    c He is under 10 years of age.
    d The mother demands a tonsillectomy.
    e The condition is preventing him from attending school.

31. Regarding quinsy, the following statements are true:
    a A quinsy is otherwise known as a peritonsillar abscess.
    b It can be treated with antibiotics and drainage.
    c It is a collection of pus outside the tonsil capsule.
    d It often occurs in patients with acute tonsillitis.
    e It is more common in children.

32. Which of the following are suggestive of a peritonsillar abscess (quinsy)?
    a Dysphagia.
    b A temperature spike.
    c Otalgia.
    d The tonsils are pushed upwards and enlarge the opening to the throat.
    e Foetor.

33. Which of the following statements are true regarding laryngotracheal trauma?
    a It must always be considered in patients with neck trauma.
    b It may present with hoarseness.
    c It should be ignored, as the larynx inevitably heals spontaneously.
    d It may present with stridor.
    e It may result in laryngeal stenosis.

34. A mother brings her ill son to see you. He has not been eating and is drooling saliva. She claims that his voice has changed and he has a fever. His sister has had flu. You notice that the boy has stridor. Which of the following statements are true regarding the management of this patient?
    a A thorough ENT clinical examination is required, including inspection of his throat.
    b The child may be sent home and the mother given advice on paracetamol administration.
    c Antibiotics are not needed, as it is most probably a viral infection.
    d The child should be given 20% oxygen using a standard mask.
    e The child should be made to cry, as this will cause vasoconstriction and relieve the neck swelling.

35. The following may be causes of acute painful dysphagia:
    a A foreign body.
    b Sinusitis.
    c Parkinson's disease.
    d Gastro-oesophageal reflux disease (GORD).
    e Tonsillitis.

36. The following are causes of chronic dysphagia:
    a An oesophageal stricture.
    b Bullous myringitis.
    c A pharyngeal pouch.
    d Globus pharyngeus.
    e Oesophageal cancer.

37. The following neurological disorders may cause dysphagia:
    a Muscular dystrophy.
    b Motor neuron disease.
    c Multiple sclerosis.
    d Alzheimer's disease.
    e Myasthenia gravis.

38. The following may be symptoms or signs of laryngeal cancer:
    a Ear pain.
    b A sore throat.
    c A hoarse voice.
    d Wheeze.
    e Right knee pain.

39. The following are symptoms of oesophageal cancer:
    a Tiredness.
    b Chest pain.
    c Dysphagia.
    d Cough.
    e Weight loss.

40. The following may be risk factors for oesophageal cancer:
    a Smoking.
    b Exposure to asbestos.
    c Barrett's oesophagus.
    d Being female.
    e A family history of the condition.

41. The following may be symptoms of oral cancer:
    a A small painless ulcer within the mouth.
    b Difficulty chewing or moving the tongue.
    c A small white patch within the mouth.
    d Sneezing.
    e Mouth pain.

42. With regard to quinsy, the following statements are true:
    a It is synonymous with the term 'retrotonsillar abscess.'
    b It is found in the nasal cavity.
    c It may deviate the uvula to the contralateral side.
    d It can present with difficulty in swallowing.
    e It is largely filled with pus.

43. A 32-year-old man has come to see you complaining of blood arising from his mouth. He has recently returned from living in South Africa for 5 years. On examination you identify a purple, friable patch on the hard palate that bleeds readily as you palpate it. The following statements may be true:
    a He has HIV.
    b This is an intraoral psoriatic plaque.
    c He has EBV.
    d This is Kaposi's sarcoma.
    e He should be isolated and quarantined.

44. The following problems may be encountered by a child with a cleft lip and palate:
   a Hearing loss.
   b Slow initial growth.
   c Speech problems.
   d Loss of the sense of smell.
   e Feeding problems.

45. The following statements are true regarding nasopharyngeal cancer:
   a It may be treated by radiotherapy.
   b It is more common in people of Afro-Caribbean origin.
   c HPV may have an important role in its aetiology.
   d It usually consists of adenocarcinomas.
   e EBV may have an important role in its aetiology.

46. The following are names of cancers found in the neck:
   a Cholesteatoma.
   b Nasal polyp.
   c Vocal cord nodule.
   d Thyroglossal cyst.
   e Quinsy.

47. You have been asked to see a young man who has fractured his jaw. Regarding mandibular fractures, the following statements are true:
   a They most commonly occur at the condyle of the mandible.
   b There may be a swelling on the floor of the mouth.
   c They may present with heightened sensation in the region of the chin.
   d They most commonly occur in the body of the mandible.
   e Most cases have more than one fracture in the mandible.

48. The following neck lumps are found in the midline of the neck:
   a Dermoid cyst.
   b Laryngocoele.
   c Thyroglossal cyst.
   d Brachial cyst.
   e Thymic cyst.

49. The following may be medical repercussions of obstructive sleep apnoea:
   a   Acromegaly.
   b   Heart failure.
   c   Asthma.
   d   Daytime somnolence.
   e   Cardiac arrhythmias.

50. The following may be symptoms of laryngeal cancer:
   a   Voice hoarseness.
   b   Haemoptysis.
   c   Ear pain.
   d   Constipation.
   e   Chest pain.

51. You are observing a panendoscopy procedure in theatre when the consultant comments that the patient has a large tongue. He subsequently asks you what the possible causes of this could be. The causes of macroglossia (a large tongue) include the following:
   a   Down syndrome.
   b   Hypothyroidism.
   c   Acromegaly.
   d   Edward's syndrome.
   e   Asthma.

52. The following cranial nerves are involved in the swallowing process:
   a   The glossopharyngeal nerve.
   b   The vestibulocochlear nerve.
   c   The vagus nerve.
   d   The abducens nerve.
   e   The radial nerve.

53. During an examination of the cranial nerves, the following clinical tests correspond to the cranial nerve cited in each case:
   a   Asking the patient to open his mouth and say 'aah' assesses the glossopharyngeal nerve.
   b   The gag reflex is innervated by the vagus nerve.
   c   Asking the patient to protrude his tongue assesses the hypoglossal nerve.
   d   Asking the patient to move his eyes up and down tests the accessory nerve.
   e   The 'jaw jerk' is innervated by the trigeminal nerve.

54. The following statements regarding laryngomalacia are true:
    a It can cause inspiratory stridor.
    b Stridor is relieved by lying the child supine and when feeding.
    c Stridor is worse on lying prone.
    d It is more common in younger children.
    e It improves as the child grows older.

55. Regarding tracheomalacia, the following statements are true:
    a It presents with inspiratory stridor.
    b It worsens with increasing age.
    c It usually affects the lower trachea.
    d The symptoms are relieved by infection.
    e It results in a higher risk of developing bronchial cancer later in
      life.

56. The following muscles are involved in swallowing:
    a Stylopharyngeus.
    b Orbicularis oculi.
    c Cricopharyngeus.
    d Rectus femoris.
    e Palatopharyngeus.

57. The following are names of the three phases of swallowing:
    a The oesophageal phase.
    b The laryngeal phase.
    c The oral phase.
    d The nasal phase.
    e The pharyngeal phase.

58. Human saliva contains the following:
    a Amylase.
    b Bicarbonate.
    c Pepsin.
    d Cholecystokinin.
    e Urobilirubin.

59. Regarding the embryological development of the larynx, which of the following statements are true?

    a The larynx descends during early childhood.
    b The arytenoid swellings begin to develop during the fourth week of gestation.
    c The larynx ascends as the child grows.
    d The arytenoid swellings develop from the sixth branchial arches.
    e The arytenoid swellings develop from mesenchymal tissue.

The throat

Answers

1. a **True.** Acid tracking up the oesophagus into the larynx can stimulate cough receptors and cause a chronic cough. The cough may improve following a course of proton pump inhibitors.
    b **True.** Patients who are taking an ACE inhibitor may also complain of a cough. This may be alleviated by replacing the medicine with an angiotensin II receptor antagonist.
    c **True.** Asthma is a cause of chronic cough. The timing of the cough should be elicited, as should any history of chest tightness or shortness of breath.
    d **True.** This is the most common cause of chronic cough. Patients may benefit from a course of antihistamines, as allergic rhinitis may be the root cause of this condition.
    e **True.** Smoking may cause a chronic cough.

2. a **True.** Some of the earliest recorded cases of this condition were congenital in origin. Congenital glottic stenosis arises from embryological failure of the larynx to form a completely patent tube, leaving webs or atresia.
    b **False.** Glottic stenosis refers to narrowing at the level of the vocal cords.
    c **True.** Intubation is a traumatic experience for the tissues of the larynx. As a result, inflammation occurs and causes fibrous tissue to start remodelling. This can result in atresia and glottic stenosis.
    d **True.** The narrowing is at the level of the vocal cords, so sound manipulation is affected. As a result, the patient may have a hoarse voice.
    e **False.** Glottic stenosis is not related to epistaxis.

3. a **True.** Vocal nodules are more common in individuals who strain their voice on a regular basis (e.g. singers).

b **True.** The presence of a vocal nodule prevents smooth closure of the vocal cords, and thus affects the sound generated.

c **False.** Vocal cord nodule surgery can result in fibrosis and subsequent distortion of the vocal cords. This will result in an irreversible voice change. It is for this reason that surgical intervention should not be chosen in the first instance. Conservative measures are the mainstay of treatment. These include advising the patient to rest his voice, as well as educating him about the condition. Irritants such as alcohol and smoking should be avoided. Surgery should be reserved for those cases that do not respond to conservative management.

d **False.** The patient should be advised to rest his voice and avoid irritants such as alcohol and smoking.

e **False.** There is no genetic inheritance of this condition. It is an acquired condition, mainly due to vocal misuse.

4. a **True.** Excess alcohol intake is a predisposing factor for the development of laryngeal cancer.

    b **False.** Like most cancers, laryngeal cancer is a disease of older patients.

    c **False.** There is no link between eating spicy food and developing laryngeal cancer. However, high intakes of dietary fats and salted meat have been indicated to be risk factors.

    d **True.** As with many other cancers, smoking is a risk factor for laryngeal cancer.

    e **True.** Men are at higher risk of developing laryngeal cancer than women.

5. a **True.** There may be difficulty in swallowing, due to the space-occupying nature of the cancer.

    b **False.** Laryngeal cancer may present with weight loss. This is partly due to the catabolic effects of the cancer itself, but is also due to the resultant dysphagia ultimately reducing food intake.

    c **True.** Feelings of fatigue and tiredness are very common in cancer. They are caused by the catabolic effects of growth of the cancer.

    d **True.** The cancer may be seen as a palpable swelling in the neck.

    e **True.** Laryngeal cancer can invoke the process of angiogenesis (the formation of new blood vessels). These blood vessels may bleed as they develop. Bleeding may also result from the effects of the cancer itself, which compresses and damages local blood vessels as it grows.

6. a **True.** Chronic tonsillitis is an indication for tonsillectomy, as is asymmetrical enlargement of the tonsils (possibly caused by a neoplasm).
    b **False.** The existence of a bleeding disorder is a contraindication for tonsillectomy, as there can be excessive blood loss during the procedure. Haemorrhage after a tonsillectomy can be divided into primary and secondary types. Primary haemorrhage occurs within 24 hours of the procedure, whereas secondary haemorrhage occurs more than 24 hours after the procedure. Secondary haemorrhage is thought to be due to infection. (This has led to many centres prescribing empirical antibiotics for secondary post-tonsillectomy haemorrhage, despite the fact that many patients lack signs of infection such as a raised temperature or pathogenic bacteria isolated by throat swabs.) Secondary post-tonsillectomy haemorrhage is currently the subject of research.
    c **True.** Obstructive sleep apnoea is an indication for tonsillectomy.
    d **False.** Obesity is also a cause of obstructive sleep apnoea, and tonsillectomy is in fact contraindicated in obese patients.
    e **True.** If more than four episodes of tonsillitis per year have a profound impact on a child's schoolwork, this is an indication for tonsillectomy. Recurrent tonsillitis secondary to a quinsy is also an indication for this surgery.

7. a **False.** Stridor and stertor sound different and have different anatomical aetiologies. Stertor sounds similar to snoring, and is an inspiratory sound originating from the upper airway, above the level of the larynx. Stridor originates from below the larynx and may be inspiratory or biphasic (both inspiratory and expiratory), depending on the location of the narrowing.
    b **False.** This statement describes stertor, not stridor. Stridor is defined as an abnormal inspiratory sound originating from below the level of the larynx, whereas stertor originates from above it.
    c **True.** This statement correctly describes stridor.
    d **False.** The type of stridor depends on the location of the airway narrowing. The typical inspiratory stridor results from narrowing just above the vocal cords. Biphasic stridor is due to narrowing either involving the vocal cords or just below them.
    e **False.** Stridor originates from the upper airways. Narrowing of the lower airways (e.g. the bronchioles) gives rise to wheezing, as in the case of asthma.

8. a **False.** Asthma is a cause of wheezing, not stridor. The best way to approach this question is to imagine the basic anatomy of the region. Stridor is caused by upper airway narrowing at or below the level of the larynx. As a result, all of the structures above the larynx and in the lower airway will not cause stridor.

b **True.** The epiglottitis is at the level of the larynx, and therefore causes stridor.

c **True.** Croup is also known as laryngotracheobronchitis. It is a viral infection that affects the upper airways of babies.

d **False.** This is a cause of stertor, as the adenoids are above the level of the larynx.

e **True.** Laryngeal cancer is a cause of stridor, as it is at the level of the larynx.

9. a **True.** The tonsils are above the level of the larynx and so result in stertor if they are enlarged. Narrowing in the upper airways at or below the level of the larynx results in stridor.

b **False.** COPD is a lower airway disease and so results in wheezing.

c **True.** The adenoids are also above the level of the larynx and so result in stertor if they are enlarged.

d **True.** Nasal obstruction is a well-documented cause of stertor.

e **False.** Acute laryngitis causes stridor, as it is at the level of the larynx.

10. a **True.** Epiglottitis is a medical emergency, so it is important to be aware of the likely causative agent when prescribing antibiotics.

b **False.** It is imperative that the child is not distressed, as this may lead to airway obstruction. Diagnosis is made on the basis of the history and from general inspection. If there is a suspicion of epiglottitis, an ENT surgeon and anaesthetist should be contacted immediately, as it is likely that the child may require intubation, or a tracheostomy in severe cases. The child should be given nebulised adrenaline and intravenous antibiotics.

c **True.** The dribbling is due to the dysphagia resulting from the swollen and inflamed epiglottis.

d **True.** The causative organism in epiglottitis is *Haemophilus influenzae* group B. The incidence of epiglottitis has been dramatically reduced by the introduction of the Hib vaccine.

e **True.** It is important to clearly recognise it and begin management immediately, as the patient can deteriorate rapidly. However, it is equally important to keep the child as relaxed as possible, as any distress may result in airway obstruction.

11. a **True.** The term laryngotracheobronchitis describes the anatomical locations involved. The term is synonymous with croup. The condition presents with a characteristic barking cough, temperature and stridor.

 b **True.** Croup is often caused by respiratory syncytial virus or parainfluenza virus.

 c **True.** Treatment is mainly supportive.

 d **False.** It is most common in young children aged between 6 months and 3 years.

 e **False.** Dangerous cases of croup may be intubated. Tracheostomy is reserved for cases where intubation has been unsuccessful.

12. a **True.** Dysphagia can be due to neurological, psychological or obstructive causes.

 b **True.** Neurological disorders may also cause dysphagia (e.g. multiple sclerosis, myasthenia gravis).

 c **False.** The vocal cords are in the larynx, and food is prevented from entering this area by the epiglottis. As a result, vocal cord nodules are not related to dysphagia (although they may cause dysphonia).

 d **True.** Thyroid cancer can grow and compress the oesophagus, resulting in dysphagia.

 e **True.** This is a functional condition in which the patient has the sensation of a lump in the throat which cannot be detected clinically or with further investigation. It is a diagnosis of exclusion.

13. a **False.** Dysphonia is the term used to describe a change in the voice. For example, a common presentation is hoarseness of the voice. Complete loss of the voice is termed aphonia.

 b **True.** Most cases of dysphonia resolve spontaneously (e.g. acute laryngitis). However, in any patient presenting with dysphonia that has lasted for more than 4 weeks, it is important to rule out cancer with an ENT referral.

 c **True.** It must be remembered that not all causes of a hoarse voice are due to vocal cord or laryngeal pathology. The vocal cords are innervated by the recurrent laryngeal nerves. These nerves branch from the vagus nerve at different points on either side. The left recurrent laryngeal nerve runs in close proximity to the left bronchus.

 d **False.** Smoking will delay recovery from dysphonia, especially in the case of laryngitis.

e **True.** Patients who frequently strain their voice (e.g. singers) are at higher risk of developing vocal cord polyps. These polyps prevent smooth adduction and closure of the vocal cords, thus causing dysphonia.

14. a **False.** Otalgia is not a complication of tracheostomy.

b **True.** Infection is an early postoperative complication.

c **True.** This is chiefly due to suturing the wound too tightly. As a result, air cannot escape and can track from the neck into the chest, resulting in surgical emphysema.

d **True.** This is more common during the operation than postoperatively.

e **True.** The tube may become blocked by tracheal secretions. However, with appropriate tube maintenance the patient will only have minimal problems.

15. a **True.** Acid can track all the way up the oesophagus and irritate the pharynx. This can present as a chronic cough, sore throat and pharyngitis.

b **True.** As with many other tissues, smoking is an irritant to the pharynx, and can induce and maintain inflammation until cessation allows time for recovery.

c **True.** Alcohol is acidic, and if consumed in large quantities over a long period of time can cause sustained inflammation of the pharynx.

d **False.** There is no association between vitamin D deficiency and chronic pharyngitis.

e **False.** There is no association between heart failure and chronic pharyngitis.

16. a **True.** These are the three stages of swallowing.

b **False.** The oral phase is under voluntary control. The other two phases are involuntary reflexes controlled by the medulla.

c **True.**

d **True.** Bulbar palsy describes impairment of the IX, X and XII cranial nerves, which results in dysphagia, dysarthria and dysphonia, respectively.

e **True.** Achalasia is an oesophageal motility disorder that results in poor peristalsis and poor relaxation of the lower sphincter, causing progressive difficulty in swallowing.

17. a **True.** Voice abuse is described as strenuous exertion of the voice. Occupations with which it is commonly associated include

singing, teaching and public speaking. Reinke's oedema is also known as bilateral diffuse polyposis. It is a swelling in the lamina propria between the vocal cord ligament and the surface epithelium (also known as Reinke's space). It responds well to conservative measures, such as smoking cessation and resting the voice.

b **False.** Epiglottitis is not related to voice abuse, and is usually caused by bacterial infection with *Haemophilus influenzae* group B.

c **True.** Vocal nodules are small nodules that usually occur on the middle third of the vocal cord. They prevent complete adduction of the cords and thus result in a hoarse voice.

d **False.** Tonsillitis is the term used to describe infection of the tonsils. It is not related to voice abuse.

e **True.** This is the formation of dilated vessels on the vocal cords. It is best treated by resting the voice and providing voice therapy.

18. a **True.** The vocal cords are the first point at which airflow starts to be shaped into sound of varying frequencies.

b **True.** The tongue and the lips are responsible for the fine manipulation of the sounds in a process called articulation.

c **True.** The teeth play a role in the finer aspects of speech articulation, as anyone who has visited an elocution teacher will know.

d **True.** As mentioned above, the lips and tongue are involved in articulation.

e **True.** Speech begins with contraction of the diaphragm. It is only after this initial flow of air that sound can be sculpted into the syllables and words that we use in everyday language. This 'sculpting' occurs in the larynx (by the vocal cords), and then in the mouth by the tongue and lips. Therefore a problem with any of these structures, their musculature or nervous supply can have a drastic impact on speech.

19. a **False.** Every physician should have a clear understanding of what to do if a patient's airway is compromised. Endotracheal intubation can offer a safe temporary airway while the required expertise is obtained. Tracheostomy is reserved for use when endotracheal intubation has failed, or if intubation is required for more than 10 days. Endotracheal intubation is otherwise quicker and safer to perform than tracheostomy, and is also associated with fewer complications.

b **False.** Children have shorter necks, which makes the insertion of a tracheostomy practically more difficult. The causes of airway obstruction in children (mainly infection) tend to resolve in a few days with antibiotic treatment, so tracheostomy is not usually necessary.

c **True.** More emergency doctors will be aware of how to intubate a patient, whereas tracheostomies are mainly performed by ENT surgeons.

d **False.** Endotracheal intubation can only safely be used for up to a maximum of 10 days, after which a tracheostomy can replace the airway.

e **True.** The endotracheal tube should be carefully inspected in case it has entered the oesophagus. Bowel sounds should be auscultated, and if there is any doubt a chest radiograph should be obtained. This complication can be fatal.

20. a **True.** The adenoids are composed of lymphatic tissue, and both the adenoids and the tonsils have roles in sleep apnoea and snoring.

b **True.** Glue ear refers to the presence of otitis media with a middle ear effusion. This can result from blockage of the Eustachian tube by the adenoids.

c **False.** Hypertrophic adenoids do not affect swallowing.

d **True.** Both of these symptoms are due to enlarged adenoids. If adenoid symptoms occur in an adult, postnasal neoplasm must be ruled out.

e **False.** Enlarged adenoids are more common in children. They grow as the child develops, and reach maximum size at around 6 years of age. They then gradually shrink to the normal size just before puberty.

21. a **True.** This is a rare condition, but is commonly asked about due to its interesting pathology. Pharyngeal pouch is a pulsion diverticulum of the pharyngeal mucosa between the upper oesophageal constrictor muscles of the cricopharyngeus and thyropharyngeus. It appears as a sac in which food and saliva may become trapped. As a result, it may present with dysphagia and cachexia.

b **True.** The sac can be palpated and may even make a gurgling sound when felt, due to food being churned inside it. This is known as Boyd's sign.

c **False.** Pharyngeal pouch is a rare disease that affects about 1 in 200 000 people each year in the UK. It is not an inherited disease, although the aetiology is not completely understood. There are several theories, including the possible influence of gastric acid refluxing up to the upper oesophageal sphincter and causing a slightly longer tonic state of muscle there. This disrupts the normal swallowing reflux, and the resulting build-up of pressure may cause minute swellings of the mucosa in the region of Killian's dehiscence, gradually forming the pouch.

d **True.** Barium swallow is the best investigation for imaging and demonstrating this pathology.

e **True.** Endoscopic surgery is the simplest, quickest and least invasive surgical intervention. However, the patient should be warned that the symptoms may not all fully resolve, but they may be greatly reduced. There is also a possibility that the pouch may reform.

22. a **True.** Angioedema can occur in anaphylaxis, and is a medical emergency. The airway can become compromised very quickly, and it is important to begin treatment immediately. Approach such a patient calmly with an ABC (Airway, Breathing and Circulation) approach initially. Inspect the patient's surroundings for a possible cause of the anaphylaxis (e.g. medication nearby), and start the patient on high-flow oxygen. It is important to memorise the following doses: 0.5 ml of 1:1000 adrenaline should be given intramuscularly in the event of angioedema formation, along with continuous blood pressure assessment. This should be preceded by 20 mg of chlorphenamine intramuscularly, and in severe cases 100 mg of hydrocortisone intramuscularly as well. These actions can prevent a fatality.

b **True.** 0.5 ml of 1:1000 adrenaline should be given intramuscularly as described above.

c **False.** Patients with angioedema should be monitored for at least 8 hours after treatment to ensure that the swelling does not return after the effects of the medication have worn off.

d **True.** Angioedema often occurs as a result of an allergy, which can be to certain medications (e.g. penicillin) or to food substances (e.g. peanuts or shellfish).

e **False.** The emergency medical measures described above resolve the majority of cases. If the airway is obstructed and does not respond to adrenaline, an emergency airway must be inserted, but this is not usually a tracheostomy.

23. a **True.** This is a flexible tube inserted through the patient's nostril down into the larynx. It is generally well tolerated, although a

local anaesthetic may be used to alleviate patient discomfort. If a local anaesthetic is used, the patient should be advised not to eat or drink for several hours after the procedure, due to the risk of aspiration. Fibre-optic nasendoscopy allows direct visualisation of the vocal cords, and is a very useful outpatient clinic investigation.

b **True.** This is a useful investigation for assessing possible causes of dysphagia. The patient swallows a solution, and a subsequent radiograph can demonstrate any abnormality, such as narrowing or a pharyngeal pouch.

c **False.** A lumbar puncture involves inserting a needle at the level of the lumbar spine in order to obtain a sample of cerebrospinal fluid for analysis. It has no role in the investigation of pathologies of the larynx or pharynx.

d **True.** Computerised tomography scanning is very useful when investigating any space-occupying lesion. It gives good resolution and an excellent indication of the relative size and location of any mass. Patients with cancers in the region of the larynx and pharynx should have a CT scan of these tumours to assess the appropriate management options.

e **False.** A D-dimer test is most commonly used to investigate the presence of a pulmonary embolism. It is not used in the investigation of the larynx or pharynx.

24. a **True.** Pooling of saliva may occur if the foreign body is obstructing the oesophagus.

b **False.** Epistaxis (bleeding from the nose) is not linked to the swallowing of a foreign body.

c **True.** The patient may be pointing to a certain region in the neck from which the pain is originating. If the pain is of sudden onset, this strongly suggests a foreign body.

d **False.** Otalgia (ear pain) is not linked to the swallowing of a foreign body.

e **False.** Coughing is a sign of an inhaled foreign body, not a swallowed foreign body.

25. a **True.** Wheezing may be present if a small foreign body has become lodged in the lower airway.

b **True.** Choking may occur if the inhaled foreign body is present in the upper airway.

c **False.** Tinnitus (hearing ringing in the ears) is not linked to the inhalation of a foreign body.

d **True.** Dyspnoea (shortness of breath) is an important sign suggestive of an inhaled foreign body. Careful and regular observations should be made of the patient's respiratory rate, pulse, oxygen saturation, blood pressure and temperature in order to assess the status of the patient. Foreign bodies that have not been identified can present with temperature and infection after some time.

e **True.** Coughing is one of the body's natural and most effective ways of clearing the upper airway of inhaled debris. This is a useful sign for distinguishing between inhaled and swallowed foreign bodies.

26. a **False.** On the basis of the patient's blue appearance, his sudden choking, and the fact that he was laughing while eating, it is most likely that he has *inhaled* a foreign body, and not swallowed it. This is a case of foreign body aspiration. It is important to differentiate swallowing from aspiration, as this will determine your next course of action. It is important to learn the management of a choking patient. An inhaled foreign body is a medical emergency which can affect anyone and can occur when least expected. Any medical practitioner should be confident in the basic emergency treatment of a choking patient.

b **True.** This is a case which would benefit from the Heimlich manoeuvre, which should be continued until the patient either recovers or becomes unconscious.

c **False.** Cardiopulmonary resuscitation (CPR) involves giving two breaths and 30 chest compressions. This is of no use in this case, as the patient's airway is blocked and no breaths will reach his lungs. Performing chest compressions will only continue to pump increasingly deoxygenated blood to the brain. The Heimlich manoeuvre is required here. This involves standing behind the patient with the patient leaning slightly forward. The physician's arms should be placed around the patient, so that the hands are clasped just below the patient's costal margin in the midline. A sudden, strong, inward and upward thrust must be made using the hands to replicate the patient's natural cough mechanism and help to clear the airway.

d **False.** Obstruction of the larynx must be cleared within a few minutes, otherwise the resulting laryngospasm will most certainly kill the patient. On the other hand, if a foreign body is obstructing one of the two bronchi, the other bronchus may still allow oxygenation of blood for a short time before the signs of hyperinflation and subsequent pneumothorax become apparent in the working lung. Any inhaled foreign body is more likely to fall into the right bronchus than the left one, as the right one is more vertical. Inhaled foreign bodies are more common in young children than in adults.

e **False.** It is highly likely that this patient may die if you do not intervene and begin the Heimlich manoeuvre.

27. a **True.** It is commonly acquired by a child at birth, from a mother who has genital warts. The result is the formation of papillomas in the child's upper airway, which may obstruct breathing as they grow.

b **True.** These are the early signs. The papillomas may later completely obstruct the airway.

c **False.** If left untreated, they will continue to increase in size. Treatment involves the use of a carbon dioxide laser in theatre.

d **True.** Therefore a child presenting with stridor or hoarseness must be investigated carefully.

e **True.** The virus is usually acquired by the neonate as it passes through the vaginal canal and comes into contact with a genital wart (caused by human papillomavirus).

28. a **False.** Globus pharyngeus (also known as globus hystericus) is the abnormal sensation of a lump in the throat. Although it is widely believed that there is a psychological element to its aetiology, studies have shown that abnormal pharyngeal motility or gastric reflux may be present in these patients.

b **False.** Some patients may benefit from antacid and reflux treatment, but ultimately reassurance is the only action indicated. Management of underlying stress or psychological issues may be discussed.

c **False.** Globus pharyngeus is most commonly a psychological condition, with no organic pathology detectable.

d **True.** Psychological conditions such as simple depression or anxiety are commonly seen in patients who present with globus pharyngeus.

e **False.** The diagnosis of globus pharyngeus is one of exclusion. Barium swallow, chest radiograph or even endoscopy may be performed to exclude organic pathology and to reassure the patient.

29. a **True.** Sleep apnoea describes transient respiratory obstruction during sleep. This results in the person waking suddenly, and can occur many times during the night. It typically presents with

daytime somnolence. Predisposing factors include those that alter the tone of the pharynx or increase the effort of breathing (e.g. the weight effects of obesity).

b **True.**

c **False.**

d **True.**

e **True.**

(now seven)

30. a **False.** Only if the patient has had more than five attacks in the last year does he qualify for a tonsillectomy. This patient has had eight attacks, and so meets these criteria. His mother also claims that he frequently has a sore throat. These may be mild cases of tonsillitis.

   b **True.** This is a requirement of the Scottish Intercollegiate Guidelines Network recommendation.

   c **False.** There is no such guidance which gives a cut-off age limit for tonsillectomy.

   d **False.** This is not a criterion for routine tonsillectomy. If the operation is not in the child's best interest, it should not proceed, no matter how demanding the mother is.

   e **True.** The recurrent tonsillitis is preventing the child from living a normal life and engaging in his usual activities.

31. a **True.**

   b **True.** Drainage can provide immediate relief.

   c **False.** Pus inside the tonsil capsule can be referred to as a quinsy.

   d **True.**

   e **False.** It is more common in adults.

32. a **True.** This is due to the resulting obstruction caused by the quinsy.

   b **True.** This is due to the infection within the quinsy.

   c **True.** This is commonly referred pain.

   d **False.** The quinsy actually forces the tonsils medially and inferiorly, which accounts for the resultant dysphagia.

   e **True.** There may be a smell emanating from the quinsy.

33. a **True.**

   b **True.** This is true for cases involving damage to the larynx.

   c **False.** It may result in an acute compromised airway, or laryngeal stenosis later on.

d **True.** This is also due to laryngeal damage, and should be investigated urgently.

e **True.** This can be prevented by early recognition and management.

34. a **False.** This boy has the characteristic signs of epiglottitis. Under no circumstances should you distress him by attempting to examine his throat until appropriate expertise and equipment have arrived to secure the airway.

    b **False.** This boy may die if you send him home. He requires admission to hospital.

    c **False.** Antibiotics should be given promptly, as epiglottitis is caused by *Haemophilus influenzae* type B.

    d **False.** 20% oxygen is less than room oxygen! The patient may require intubation, as the epiglottitis may be preventing air from reaching the lungs.

    e **False.** Under no circumstances whatsoever should the child be distressed, as this could trigger a potentially fatal airway obstruction. The child should be kept calm until the appropriate expertise arrives.

35. a **True.** A foreign body is an important differential diagnosis to consider in any patient who is complaining of sudden-onset painful dysphagia.

    b **False.** Sinusitis does not cause dysphagia.

    c **False.** Parkinson's disease is caused by degeneration of dopaminergic pathways in the substantia nigra. It is characterised by the triad of rigidity, resting tremor and slowness of movement. It is not a cause of acute, painful dysphagia. Most neurological causes of dysphagia do not tend to be painful, and their onset is more gradual in nature (except for stroke).

    d **True.** Gastric acid refluxing up the oesophagus can cause irritation and tonic activity in the pharynx. This can lead to dysphagia.

    e **True.** Tonsillitis can also cause painful dysphagia as the swollen and inflamed tissue is disturbed on swallowing.

36. a **True.** Structural and anatomical obstructions in the food passage are an important cause of long-term dysphagia.

    b **False.** This is a condition in which abnormal vesicles appear on the tympanic membrane in the ear. It is not related to dysphagia.

    c **True.** This abnormal outpouching of the pharyngeal mucosa is a rare but debilitating cause of dysphagia.

d **True.** This condition can be a source of frustration for clinicians. No structural explanation for the dysphagia can be found, and it is thought to be primarily a psychological condition. Enquiry into life stresses and problems can elucidate a potential psychosomatic element to the disease, and treatment may involve addressing underlying social issues.

e **True.** Oesophageal cancer is a difficult cancer to treat, and the dysphagia that it causes can result in rapid weight loss due to both lack of nutrition and the catabolic effects of the cancer itself.

37. a **True.** Oculopharyngeal muscular dystrophy presents after around 50 years of age, and the patient may have difficulty in swallowing both solids and liquids. Not all causes of dysphagia are structural, and although neuromuscular causes of dysphagia fall within the remit of neurologists, it is important to be aware of the various signs and symptoms, so that the patient can be referred to the appropriate specialty.

b **True.** There are various forms of motor neuron disease, and they all result in dysphagia to varying degrees.

c **True.** Multiple sclerosis is caused by demyelination of central neurons. This results in a number of symptoms, including dysphagia.

d **False.** Alzheimer's disease mainly affects the memory and cognition. It does not cause dysphagia.

e **True.** This is an autoimmune condition in which antibodies to post-synaptic acetylcholine receptors reduce neuronal transmission. The result is an excessive weakness, and fatiguability in muscles as they are used.

38. a **True.** Referred ear pain can originate from the larynx. This is a very important point to remember when examining any patient who presents with otalgia.

b **True.** Neck pain can be a sign of laryngeal cancer.

c **True.** If any patient has had a hoarse voice for more than 3 weeks, they should be referred to an ENT department.

d **False.** Wheezing occurs as a result of narrowing of the lower airway tract. Laryngeal cancer causes narrowing higher in the respiratory tract, and gives rise to inspiratory stridor.

e **False.** Laryngeal cancer does not directly cause knee pain.

39. a **True.** Tiredness is due to both malnutrition and the cancer itself.

b **True.** Chest pain arises from the space-occupying effects of the cancer.

  c **True.** Dysphagia is due to narrowing of the food passage as the cancer increases in size.

  d **False.** Cough is not a common symptom of oesophageal cancer.

  e **True.** Weight loss is due both to malnutrition and to the catabolic effects of the cancer itself.

40. a **True.** The various carcinogens in cigarette smoke make it a risk factor for oesophageal cancer.

     b **False.** Asbestos exposure can give rise to mesothelioma in the lungs, but not to oesophageal cancer.

     c **True.** Barrett's oesophagus is the abnormal metaplasia of squamous epithelium into columnar epithelium at the lower end of the oesophagus, due to gastro-oesophageal reflux. The condition is a risk factor for the development of oesophageal cancer.

     d **False.** Men are at higher risk of developing oesophageal cancer than women.

     e **True.** A family history of oesophageal cancer is a risk factor for developing the disease.

41. a **True.** This can be the initial appearance of oral cancers, and is more suspicious if it does not heal within a couple of weeks.

     b **True.** The growth of a cancer distorts the natural concaves of the mouth. As a result, it can present with difficulties in chewing and moving the tongue.

     c **True.** This is called leukoplakia, and it is a pre-malignant condition.

     d **False.** Sneezing is not a symptom of oral cancers.

     e **True.** Oral cancer can be painful, but this is a late sign.

42. a **False.** It is synonymous with the term 'peritonsillar abscess', not 'retrotonsillar abscess.'

     b **False.** Quinsies are found at the back of the throat on either side of the uvula along the tonsils.

     c **True.** A quinsy grows as it swells with pus. This space-occupying effect can push the uvula away from it towards the opposite side.

     d **True.** Quinsies typically cause pain and difficulty in swallowing and speaking.

     e **True.** In the treatment of quinsies, a needle or fine scalpel can be used to drain the pus. This may alleviate many of the patient's symptoms. It is important to ask when the patient ate their last meal, as a local anaesthetic spray is used during the procedure, and it can disrupt the swallowing process.

43. a **True.** This patient has Kaposi's sarcoma, which can occur in HIV-positive patients.
    b **False.** Psoriasis does not affect the lining of the mouth.
    c **False.** Epstein–Barr virus does not cause this type of lesion within the mouth.
    d **True.** The description of the lesion is strongly suggestive of Kaposi's sarcoma. In addition, the patient has returned from a country where there are high rates of HIV in some regions.
    e **False.** This patient has HIV, as Kaposi's sarcoma is an AIDS-defining lesion. He should receive the relevant counselling, and informed consent should be obtained to investigate and treat him. He should have a blood test to assess his CD4 count, and should be started on an appropriate antiretroviral treatment as soon as possible. HIV patients are not quarantined, but education about the disease must be provided.

44. a **True.** Conductive hearing loss results from distortion of the Eustachian tube anatomy. As a result, these children are at greater risk of developing glue ear.
    b **True.** This is usually due to poor feeding if the child is breastfed. The cleft lip affects the child's suckling, and so may prevent him from gaining the optimum nutrition that he needs in order to grow.
    c **True.** Patients with a cleft lip and palate will have more nasal-sounding speech than other children. Surgical repair of this condition can also result in abnormal speech as a complication.
    d **False.** Children with a cleft lip and palate have a normal sense of smell.
    e **True.** These children have difficulty breastfeeding and have unusual tooth development later.

45. a **True.** Radiotherapy is an effective treatment modality for nasopharyngeal cancers, especially when combined with concurrent chemotherapy in eligible patients.
    b **False.** It is more common in people from China and south-east Asia.
    c **False.** Human papillomavirus is associated with laryngeal cancer.
    d **False.** They are usually squamous-cell cancers.
    e **True.** Epstein–Barr virus is associated with nasopharyngeal cancers.

46. a **False.** Cholesteatoma is found in the ear canal, not the neck. A cholesteatoma is a benign growth. It is not considered to be a

cancer and does not metastasise. However, if untreated it can go on to cause devastating damage to surrounding structures as it increases in size.

b **False.** Nasal polyps are not like colorectal polyps and do not indicate the possibility of cancer.

c **False.** In any patient who presents with dysphonia it is vital to exclude cancer. Vocal cord nodules are calluses on the vocal cord and are not considered to be cancers.

d **False.** This is a congenital remnant and is not a cancer.

e **False.** A quinsy is a peritonsillar abscess, not a cancer. The main message behind this question is that not all enlarging masses or lumps are cancers. However, they should only be diagnosed after cancer has been excluded.

47. a **False.** They are actually less common in the mandibular condyle. They most often occur in the body of the mandible.

b **True.** A swelling may reflect haematoma formation as a result of the mandibular fracture.

c **False.** They may have accompanying numbness and loss of sensation in the region of the chin, due to damage to the inferior alveolar nerve.

d **True.** Mandibular fractures most commonly occur in the body of the mandible.

e **True.** The ring formed by the mandible means that any force will be distributed across the bone. Subsequently, mandibular fractures rarely occur singly. There are commonly two or more fractures, usually at opposing points on the bone.

48. a **True.** This congenital lump can be found in the midline, and may contain any number of different tissues.

b **False.** This outpouching of the laryngeal mucosa is most often seen in wind instrument players, as blowing creates high pressures within the larynx. This results in the protrusion and formation of the laryngocoele. It is usually found lateral to the midline.

c **True.** This congenital lump is seen in the midline, and it rises on protrusion of the tongue.

d **False.** A branchial cyst is a congenital remnant that is found lateral to the midline.

e **True.** Thymic cysts are often found in the midline.

49. a **False.** Acromegaly is an endocrine disorder and is not caused by obstructive sleep apnoea (although acromegalic patients may suffer from that condition).

   b **True.** Both left and right heart failure can develop as a result of the effects of obstructive sleep apnoea.

   c **False.** Asthma has a complex aetiology but is not caused by obstructive sleep apnoea.

   d **True.** Sleepiness or personality changes during the day are the direct results of sleep deprivation due to obstructive sleep apnoea.

   e **True.** Arrhythmias are widely known to develop from hypoxic states. As a result, obstructive sleep apnoea is a risk factor for cardiac arrhythmias.

50. a **True.** A patient who presents with a prolonged cough or voice change should be referred for investigation. Hoarseness of the voice is a feature of laryngeal cancer.

   b **True.** Patients with laryngeal cancer may cough up blood. This is partly due to the angiogenesis of the cancer.

   c **True.** Referred pain to the ear can occur in patients with laryngeal cancer.

   d **False.** Constipation is not a feature of laryngeal cancer.

   e **False.** Chest pain is not a feature of laryngeal cancer, although neck or throat pain may occur.

51. a **True.** Down syndrome is caused by a chromosomal abnormality (trisomy 21). It has various signs, including macroglossia.

   b **True.** Macroglossia is a feature of hypothyroidism.

   c **True.** Macroglossia is a feature of acromegaly.

   d **False.** Edward's syndrome is caused by a chromosomal abnormality (trisomy 18). It is not associated with macroglossia.

   e **False.** There is no link between asthma and macroglossia.

52. a **True.** The glossopharyngeal nerve supplies pharyngeal sensation and innervates the stylopharyngeus. This nerve is involved in the swallowing process.

   b **False.** The vestibulocochlear nerve is responsible for hearing and balance. It does not have a direct role in the swallowing process.

   c **True.** The vagus nerve is involved in the swallowing process. A lesion of this nerve will result in dysphagia due to palatal and pharyngeal paralysis.

    d **False.** The abducens nerve is the sixth cranial nerve and it innervates the lateral rectus muscle. It does not have a role in swallowing.

    e **False.** The radial nerve is not a cranial nerve. It is supplied by the nerve roots C5–T1 and innervates the muscles on the extensor aspect of the upper limb. It also has a small sensory component in the upper limb.

53. a **True.** Asking the patient to open his mouth and say 'aah' allows assessment of the uvula and palate movement. This test examines both the glossopharyngeal and vagus nerve. The 'gag' reflex can be elicited in order to further assess these cranial nerves.

    b **True.** The glossopharyngeal nerve supplies the sensory aspect of this reflex, and the actual motor response is innervated by the vagus nerve.

    c **True.** The hypoglossal nerve innervates the tongue. Any deviation of the tongue should be carefully inspected, and speech can be assessed by asking the patient to say 'yellow lorry.'

    d **False.** The accessory nerve innervates the sternocleidomastoid and part of the trapezius muscle. It is tested by asking the patient to move their from head side to side and shrug their shoulders against resistance.

    e **True.** The 'jaw jerk' can be elicited by gently tapping a tendon hammer downward at the chin with the mouth relaxed in a slightly open position. The masseter muscle is responsible for a reflex closing of the mouth in response to this stimulus. The trigeminal nerve innervates this reflex.

54. a **True.** Laryngomalacia is a cause of inspiratory stridor.

    b **False.** The stridor of a child who is suffering from laryngomalacia is worse on lying supine and during feeding. It is characteristically relieved by positioning the child so that they are lying prone.

    c **False.** The stridor of a child who is suffering from laryngomalacia is actually relieved by positioning the child so that they are lying prone.

    d **True.** Laryngomalacia is particularly common in neonates and young children.

    e **True.** Laryngomalacia is caused by the soft supporting cartilage that is found in these children. As the child grows, the cartilage stiffens and the symptoms resolve.

55. a **False.** Unlike laryngomalacia, which presents with inspiratory stridor, tracheomalacia presents with expiratory stridor.

b **False.** The pathophysiology of tracheomalacia is similar to that of laryngomalacia. Tracheomalacia is also caused by soft, flaccid cartilage, so the symptoms resolve as the child grows and the cartilage hardens.

c **True.** Tracheomalacia usually affects the lower part of the trachea.

d **False.** The symptoms of tracheomalacia are exacerbated by infection.

e **False.** There is no association between tracheomalacia and bronchial cancer.

56. a **True.** The stylopharyngeus muscle links the styloid process and the pharynx. It functions to raise the larynx upward and forward during swallowing.

b **False.** The orbicularis oculi muscle is responsible for closing the eye. This muscle has no role in the swallowing process.

c **True.** The cricopharyngeus muscle plays an important role in the functioning of the upper oesophageal sphincter. The vagus nerve holds it in a tonically constricted state before swallowing.

d **False.** The rectus femoris is part of the quadriceps group of muscles. It has no role in swallowing.

e **True.** The palatopharyngeus muscle aids the movement of the bolus into the lower pharynx.

57. a **True.** The oesophageal phase is in fact the third and final phase of the swallowing process. It involves the movement of the bolus down the oesophagus to the stomach via a peristaltic oesophageal muscle contraction.

b **False.** The food should never enter the larynx, so there should never be a laryngeal phase! The epiglottis is responsible for folding over the larynx and preventing food from entering it during the pharyngeal phase of swallowing. If food enters the larynx there is a risk of aspiration pneumonia.

c **True.** The oral phase is the first stage of swallowing, and involves the mastication of food and subsequent formation of a bolus. The bolus is moved to the back of the throat, and this stage ends when the bolus reaches the anterior faucial arches. It is here that the pharyngeal stage begins.

d **False.** The food should not enter the nasal cavity! There is no 'nasal phase' in the normal swallowing process.

e **True.** The pharyngeal stage of swallowing is the second step in the process. During this stage the bolus is moved into the laryngopharynx and various protective mechanisms come into play, such as closing of the epiglottis. The oesophageal stage follows this step.

58. a **True.** Amylase is an enzyme involved in the digestion of starch. It works most effectively at a slightly alkaline pH, and therefore becomes active as soon as the food enters the mouth.

b **True.** Bicarbonate has an important role in regulating the pH so that it is at the optimum value for salivary amylase to work.

c **False.** Pepsin is an enzyme involved in the digestion of proteins. It is active at an acidic pH, and is produced by the chief cells in the stomach.

d **False.** Cholecystokinin is a hormone produced by the duodenum, and it acts on the gallbladder and pancreas.

e **False.** Urobilirubin is a product of the hepatic metabolism of bilirubin. It is further oxidised and excreted by the kidneys, and is responsible for the colour of urine.

59. a **True.** The larynx actually moves inferiorly from its position at birth (C1–C4) to its mature position (between the C4 and C7 vertebrae). This movement coincides with the development of increasing fine vocalisation.

b **True.**

c **False.** The larynx descends in early childhood.

d **True.** The sixth branchial arch gives rise to all of the intrinsic muscles of the larynx (except the cricothyroid muscle and the arytenoid and cricoid cartilage). It also gives rise to the recurrent laryngeal nerve (which innervates the vocal cords).

e **True.** Mesenchymal tissue is a form of loose connective tissue that can develop into a wide range of specialised tissues, including cartilage, bone and lymphatic tissue. It is the embryological tissue derivative of the arytenoid cartilage.

Head and neck surgery

Questions

1. Regarding nasopharyngeal carcinoma, the following statements are true:
   a It is more common in people of Chinese origin.
   b It is a columnar-cell cancer.
   c It may present with epistaxis.
   d A fibre-optic nasoendoscope may allow visualisation of the cancer.
   e With treatment, the average survival rate at 5 years is 5%.

2. Which of the following factors affect the prognosis of a head and neck cancer?
   a Its size.
   b Its histological cell type.
   c Its colour.
   d The involvement of lymph nodes.
   e The patient's age and general health.

3. The following are risk factors for head and neck cancer:
   a Radiation exposure.
   b Smoking.
   c Eating sugary foods.
   d Genetics.
   e Alcohol.

4. Which of the following statements are true regarding head and neck cancers?
   a They are most aggressive in children, and commonly form distant metastases quickly.
   b If a palpable lump is present, fine-needle aspiration (FNA) should be performed for histological analysis.
   c Lymphadenopathy must always be palpated for.
   d The location of the lump with regard to the triangles in the neck can aid the differential diagnosis.
   e Head and neck cancers are always primary cancers.

5. Regarding dermoid cysts, which of the following statements are true?
   a They are usually present just below the chin in the midline.
   b They are lined with epithelium.
   c They may contain teeth, nails or hair.
   d They move up on swallowing.
   e They are an acquired condition.

6. Regarding pharyngeal cancer, which of the following statements are true?
   a It is more common in young girls who are non-smokers.
   b This is a squamous-cell cancer.
   c It may present with throat pain.
   d It can be investigated by MRI.
   e It can be managed by surgery.

7. A patient presents with a unilateral lump in the region of the parotid gland. Which of the following statements are true regarding parotid tumours?
   a The vast majority of these tumours are pleomorphic adenomas.
   b The trigeminal nerve may be affected by the growth of a parotid lump, leading to reduced facial expression on that side.
   c They may be treated by performing a superficial parotidectomy.
   d After surgery, some patients may sweat on the operated side of the face while eating.
   e A fine-needle aspiration should not be performed, as this may well spread the cancer.

8. The following structures make up the borders of the anterior trian-
    gle of the neck:
    a The posterior border of the sternocleidomastoid muscle.
    b The inferior border of the mandible.
    c The anterior border of the sternocleidomastoid muscle.
    d The anterior aspect of the trapezius muscle.
    e The midline of the neck.

9. The following may be lumps found in the anterior triangle of the
    neck:
    a Parotid tumour.
    b Carotid body tumour.
    c Laryngocoele.
    d Cervical rib.
    e Cystic hygroma.

10. Regarding oral cancers:
    a The tongue is most affected.
    b They are usually transitional-cell carcinomas.
    c They may appear like an ulcer.
    d Smoking is a risk factor.
    e Leukoplakia is a premalignant condition.

11. The following are types of thyroid cancer:
    a Follicular.
    b Medullary.
    c Sponge idiopathic.
    d Anaplastic.
    e Papillary.

12. The following are signs or symptoms of hyperthyroidism:
    a Anxiety and agitation.
    b Sweating.
    c Tremor.
    d Weight gain
    e Bradycardia.

13. The following are signs or symptoms of hypothyroidism:
    a Loss of hair from the lateral third of the eyebrow.
    b Lethargy and fatigue.
    c Diarrhoea.
    d Concentration difficulty.
    e Depression.

14. You have been asked to see a patient with a low calcium level. She has recently had a total thyroidectomy. Which of the following signs would you look for to suggest hypocalcaemia?
    a Trousseau sign.
    b Chvostek's sign.
    c De Musset's sign.
    d Pistol-shot femoral pulse sounds.
    e Carpopedal spasm.

15. A patient has presented with symptoms of hyperthyroidism and an enlarged thyroid. You send off a blood sample for thyroid function tests. Which of the following results would best support your diagnosis?
    a A high TSH level.
    b A low TSH level.
    c A high T3 level.
    d A low T3 level.
    e A low alanine transferase level.

16. Regarding primary hyperparathyroidism, which of the following statements are true?
    a It causes hypocalcaemia.
    b It is usually due to a lone adenoma.
    c It is common in children.
    d It is always due to invasive cancer.
    e It is due to excess thyroid-stimulating hormone.

17. Regarding papillary thyroid cancer, which of the following statements are true?
    a It is the most common of all the thyroid cancers.
    b It may be spread by fine-needle aspiration.
    c First-line treatment is chemotherapy.
    d It has a good prognosis.
    e It is more common in men.

18. Regarding follicular thyroid cancer, which of the following statements are true?
    a It is more common in children.
    b It is more common in women.
    c It cannot be treated surgically.
    d It has a better prognosis if it is larger in size.
    e It is the rarest thyroid cancer.

19. Regarding medullary thyroid cancer, which of the following statements are true?
    a It is more common in middle-aged patients.
    b It can be part of multiple endocrine neoplasia (MEN) syndrome.
    c It is an aggressive and fast-growing cancer.
    d It can metastasise to the liver.
    e Around 25% of cases are familial in nature.

20. Regarding anaplastic thyroid cancer, which of the following statements are true?
    a It may arise from papillary thyroid cancer.
    b It is a slow-growing cancer.
    c It rarely metastasises.
    d It is treated by thyroidectomy.
    e It has a good prognosis.

21. You have been asked by your registrar to consent a patient for a thyroidectomy operation. The following may be possible complications of surgery that the patient should be aware of:
    a Vocal cord paralysis.
    b Haematoma formation.
    c Epistaxis.
    d Hypocalcaemia.
    e Infection.

22. Regarding basal-cell cancer, which of the following statements are true?
    a They are fast-growing cancers.
    b They most commonly occur in light-skinned, Caucasian patients.
    c They are the most common skin cancer.
    d They commonly metastasise to other areas of the body.
    e Solar keratosis is the premalignant form.

23. Regarding melanoma, which of the following statements are true?
    a It may be classified using Clark's classification.
    b If resected, it requires a 50 mm margin.
    c It may be classified using Breslow thickness.
    d If lymph nodes are positive, a neck dissection is required.
    e A positive family history is a risk factor.

24. Regarding the TNM cancer staging system:
    a 'T' refers to 'tumour' and scores the size of the tumour on a scale of 1–4.
    b 'N' refers to the number of lymph nodes involved.
    c 'N' refers to the size of the lymph nodes involved.
    d 'N' is scored on a scale of 0–3.
    e 'M' refers to 'metastasis' and is scored on a scale of 0–5.

25. The larynx has the following roles:
    a Prevention of aspiration.
    b Phonation.
    c Odour sensation.
    d Coughing.
    e Proprioception.

26. Regarding acute sialadenitis, which of the following statements are true?
    a It is inflammation of the salivary glands.
    b It presents with redness, swelling and pain over the gland.
    c It is caused by stasis of saliva.
    d It is commonly caused by listeria meningitis.
    e It may be relieved by gentle massage of the gland.

27. The following are the names of salivary glands in the head and neck:
    a Parotid gland.
    b Lacrimal gland.
    c Sublingual gland.
    d Submandibular gland.
    e Pituitary gland.

28. Regarding salivary calculi, which of the following statements are true?
    a They most commonly occur in the parotid gland.
    b They can result in sialadenitis.
    c They may result in gland swelling during meals.
    d They are improved by dehydration.
    e Gout has a preventative effect.

29. A 5-year-old boy presents with bilateral gland swelling. He has a sore throat and fever. His mother explains that he has been tired and complains of pain in his cheeks. She admits that she did *not* give consent for him to have the MMR vaccine, due to fears about autism. Which of the following statements are true?
    a This child has bilateral salivary calculi.
    b He urgently requires antibiotics.
    c This condition could have been prevented by the MMR vaccine.
    d The child should have a hearing test when he is more stable.
    e His condition could be potentially fatal.

30. Regarding Sjögren's syndrome, which of the following statements are true?
    a It is a systemic autoimmune disorder.
    b It may present with excessive tear and saliva production.
    c Treatment may involve prescription of artificial tear drops.
    d Antibody tests are negative for anti-nuclear antibody and rheumatoid factor.
    e Schirmer's test is usually negative.

31. Complications of a parotidectomy include the following:
    a Damage to the facial nerve.
    b Frey's syndrome.
    c Greater auricular nerve damage.
    d Damage to the vestibulocochlear nerve.
    e Infection.

32. The following are eye signs of thyroid disease:
    a Exophthalmos.
    b Lid lag.
    c Lid retraction.
    d Ophthalmoplegia.
    e Presbyopia.

33. The following are possible complications of a total laryngectomy:
    a Voice change.
    b Pharyngeal stenosis.
    c Sensorineural hearing loss.
    d Aspiration pneumonia.
    e Chronic sinusitis.

34. The following are the names of groups of lymph nodes in the head and neck:
    a Occipital.
    b Orbital.
    c Tracheal.
    d Mastoid.
    e Deep cervical.

35. For a patient suffering from voice loss following a total laryngectomy, the following methods of communication are available:
    a Gastro-oesophageal speech.
    b Tracheo-oesophageal fistula.
    c Sign language.
    d Artificial voice generators.
    e Eye contact.

36. Regarding laryngeal cancer, which of the following statements are true?
    a It most commonly occurs in the glottis.
    b It may present with voice hoarseness.
    c It is commonly a squamous-cell cancer.
    d It is a benign condition.
    e The prognosis depends upon which part of the larynx is affected.

37. The following are chemotherapy agents used in head and neck cancer:
    a 5-Fluorouracil.
    b Tramadol.
    c Metronidazole.
    d Cisplatin.
    e Methotrexate.

38. The following are possible presentations of carotid body tumours:
    a Horner's syndrome.
    b Tongue weakness.
    c Pain.
    d Voice hoarseness.
    e Anterior triangle neck lump.

39. Regarding Bell's palsy, which of the following statements are true?
    a Vesicles may be visible in the auditory canal.
    b It affects the seventh cranial nerve.
    c It can present with drooping of the corner of the mouth.
    d It may be caused by Epstein–Barr virus.
    e It may cause weakness on one side of the face.

40. The following are branches of the facial nerve:
    a Cervical.
    b Temporal.
    c Zygomatic.
    d Maxillary.
    e Buccal.

41. Regarding sinus cancer, which of the following statements are true?
    a It can be detected early in the disease.
    b A skull radiograph should be performed to visualise the cancer.
    c It may present with epistaxis.
    d It most commonly occurs in the maxillary sinus.
    e It is most commonly a squamous-cell cancer.

42. The following are the names of sinuses in the head:
    a Ethmoidal.
    b Frontal.
    c Maxillary.
    d Mandibular.
    e Sphenoidal.

43. The following are parts of the pharynx:
    a Larynx.
    b Oropharynx.
    c Laryngopharynx.
    d Nasopharynx.
    e Sinupharynx.

44. The facial nerve supplies innervation to the following glands:
    a Lacrimal gland.
    b Sublingual gland.
    c Parotid gland.
    d Submandibular gland.
    e Pituitary gland.

45. With regard to the salivary glands, which of the following statements are true?
    a There are three paired major salivary glands, namely the parotid gland, submandibular gland and sublingual gland.
    b Parasympathetic innervation causes salivary secretion.
    c The glossopharyngeal nerve innervates the parotid gland.
    d The facial nerve passes through the parotid gland and splits into its five main divisions.
    e The saliva produced is strongly acidic.

46. Regarding sialadenitis, which of the following statements are true?
    a The term describes inflammation of a salivary gland.
    b It usually occurs in children.
    c Poor oral hygiene is one of the contributing factors.
    d It can result in painful swallowing.
    e It is usually treated with antibiotics and rehydration if applicable.

47. Regarding sialolithiasis (salivary stones), which of the following statements are true?
    a It commonly affects the submandibular gland.
    b It classically presents as pain on eating, accompanied by swelling of the affected gland.
    c Plain radiograph or sialography confirms the presence of salivary stones.
    d Salivary stones must be removed surgically.
    e The affected gland may need to be removed if the stone does not pass.

48. With regard to salivary gland tumours, which of the following statements are true?
    a They most commonly occur in the submandibular gland.
    b Around 50% of the tumours that occur in the submandibular gland are malignant.
    c Facial nerve paresis could suggest malignancy.
    d It is difficult to differentiate between benign and malignant salivary gland tumours on the basis of symptoms alone.
    e Tumours of the minor salivary glands are usually benign.

49. Regarding the embryological development of the head and neck, which of the following structures are derived from the first pharyngeal arch?
    a The masseter muscle.
    b The maxilla.
    c The temporalis muscle.
    d The mandible.
    e The orbicularis oris muscle.

50. The following statements regarding buccal carcinoma are true:
    a These cancers tend to reoccur.
    b Alcohol is a risk factor.
    c They can be treated surgically.
    d Epstein–Barr virus infection is a risk factor.
    e They are most commonly of squamous-cell origin.

51. The following statements regarding oral tongue cancer are true:
    a It is most commonly of columnar-cell origin.
    b Surgical treatment may result in altered speech.
    c Smoking has a protective effective effect on this type of cancer.
    d It may be treated by a gastrectomy.
    e It can affect swallowing.

52. During a radical neck dissection, the following structures are most commonly excised:
    a The platysma muscle.
    b The common carotid artery.
    c The omohyoid muscle.
    d The vagus nerve.
    e The phrenic nerve.

53. The following muscles are supplied by the ansa cervicalis:
    a Sternohyoid.
    b Sternothyroid.
    c Pectoralis major.
    d Sternocleidomastoid.
    e Omohyoid.

54. With regard to conditions of the head and neck, the following statements are true:
    a Persistent unilateral otalgia could denote an occult throat tumour.
    b A patient with a persistent change in voice should be referred for speech therapy as a first step.
    c A patient with a neck lump should be referred to a general or vascular surgeon for a diagnostic incisional or excisional biopsy.
    d The single most useful investigation for a neck lump is a fine-needle aspiration biopsy.
    e The first investigation for a neck lump should be a CT scan of the neck, chest, abdomen and pelvis to rule out lymphoma.

Head and neck surgery

Answers

1. a **True.** Nasopharyngeal carcinoma is more common in people of Chinese origin, for a number of possible reasons. A diet of salted fish in early childhood may be a contributing factor (due to the N-nitroso carcinogens that it contains). Infection with Epstein–Barr virus may also increase the risk of developing this cancer. Genetic predisposition is an important factor in all cancers, and certain alleles are more prevalent in the Chinese population than in other ethnic subgroups. The higher numbers of smokers in China compared with western countries may also be a contributing factor.

   b **False.** It is a squamous-cell cancer (which may or may not be keratinising), but may include transitional-cell carcinomas, lymphoepitheliomas and angiofibromas.

   c **True.** Nasopharyngeal carcinoma can present with nasal obstruction and epistaxis. It may grow to impact on the cranial nerves and result in their respective palsies. The space-occupying effect of the tumour may block the Eustachian tube and thus result in a middle ear effusion and subsequent conductive hearing loss.

   d **True.** This is a simple outpatients clinic procedure that involves inserting a flexible tube into the nose. The tube has a camera at one end and can allow the examiner to see the nasal passage in more detail. It is also possible to obtain biopsies using a similar device.

   e **False.** The prognosis of the patient depends on their age and health, the staging of the cancer, and the management plan that is devised. Radiotherapy is the main treatment modality. However, surgery and chemotherapy may also be incorporated into the management plan. Nasopharyngeal carcinoma has a relatively good prognosis, certainly not as low as that stated in the question. Patients have a 40–60% survival rate at 5 years, depending on the staging.

2. a **True.** There are many staging pro formas available. However, the TNM system is widely accepted.

    b **True.** This is obtained by a biopsy of the cancer and it yields important prognostic information. Some cell types grow more aggressively than others, and are more likely to spread and metastasise.

    c **False.** The 'colour' of the tumour does not affect the prognosis.

    d **True.** This suggests spread and metastasis of the cancer.

    e **True.** The patient's general health indicates how much reserve they will have when faced with the cancer process and the possible treatment.

3. a **True.** To answer this question you must apply your general knowledge of all cancers. Exposure to radiation is a risk factor for all cancers, as it induces mutations at the genetic level.

    b **True.** Cigarette smoke contains a number of toxic and carcinogenic compounds, and the mouth and throat are the sites of first contact with this hazardous cocktail of gases.

    c **False.** There is no link between eating sugary food and developing head and neck cancer. However, such a diet may cause problems of its own (e.g. diabetes mellitus).

    d **True.** Some people are more likely to develop a head and neck cancer than others, by virtue of their genetic make-up. Some individuals may even have genetic syndromes (e.g. MEN syndrome) that predispose them to a number of different cancers.

    e **True.** Like smoking, alcohol is a potential carcinogen if consumed excessively over a long period of time.

4. a **False.** Fortunately, head and neck neoplasms in children are usually benign. However, in adults they are more likely to become malignant.

    b **True.** FNA allows analysis of the constituent cell types. This is very useful when determining the primary site of cancer, as well as for staging the cancer for prognosis.

    c **True.** Enlarged lymph nodes may be a sign that the cancer has metastasised, and must not be omitted during examination.

    d **True.** A basic anatomical understanding of the various glands and structures in each neck triangle can help you to narrow down what a lump could be.

    e **False.** A primary cancer is one that has originated at the site where it has been discovered. A secondary cancer is one that has metastasised (to the site where it has been discovered) from its origin in a different part of the body. Some head and neck tumours are secondary cancers from the stomach, kidney, prostate, breast, uterus, pancreas or lung.

5. a **True.** Dermoid cysts present considerably higher up than the usual location of a thyroglossal cyst. They are usually excised.
    b **True.**
    c **True.** The tissue contained in these cysts is a remnant of embryological development, so it is not uncommon to find hair or teeth within dermoid cysts.
    d **False.** Thyroglossal cysts move up on swallowing, but dermoid cysts do not.
    e **False.** Dermoid cysts are formed during embryological development and are a congenital condition, not an acquired one.

6. a **False.** This cancer is more common in elderly male smokers.
    b **True.** The vast majority are squamous-cell cancers.
    c **True.** Patients with pharyngeal cancer may present with throat pain, dysphagia and voice change.
    d **True.** Magnetic resonance imaging (MRI) makes it possible to ascertain the size of the cancer, as well as its relationship to the surrounding anatomical structures.
    e **True.** Management of the pharyngeal cancer involves surgical resection. However, if the cancer is small, radiotherapy may be used as first-line treatment.

7. a **True.** Pleomorphic adenoma is usually a benign tumour, and is one of the most commonly occurring parotid gland lumps.
    b **False.** It is the facial nerve which has an intimate relationship with the parotid gland. The trigeminal nerve innervates the sensory neurons in the face and the muscles of mastication. The facial nerve is responsible for the muscles of facial expression.
    c **True.** Parotid tumours may occasionally be treated by performing a superficial parotidectomy. The facial nerve is sometimes affected during surgery, leading to drooping of that side of the face. This may be transient and the patient may recover, but occasionally the drooping is permanent.
    d **True.** As unlikely as this may sound, it is a recognised complication of parotid surgery. It is called Frey's syndrome, and is due to inappropriate innervation of the sweat glands during the healing process after surgery. It is also known as 'gustatory sweating.'

e **False.** Fine-needle aspiration does not result in 'seeding', or spread of the cancer. It is an important and prognostically significant investigation that is very safe in skilled hands.

8. a **False.** Remember to read the question carefully. This question is asking for the names of the structures that make up the borders of the *anterior* triangle of the neck. The posterior border of the sternocleidomastoid muscle is part of the posterior triangle of the neck. It is the anterior border of the sternocleidomastoid that demarcates the anterior triangle.
   b **True.** The inferior border of the mandible marks the superior aspect of the anterior triangle.
   c **True.** The anterior border of the sternocleidomastoid muscle marks the lateral border of the anterior triangle.
   d **False.** The anterior aspect of the trapezius muscle marks the lateral border of the posterior triangle, not of the anterior triangle.
   e **True.** The midline of the neck marks the medial aspect of the anterior triangle.

9. a **True.** A parotid tumour can grow inferiorly.
   b **True.** The carotid pulses can be felt in the anterior triangle. A carotid body tumour is called a chemodectoma, and may be seen in the anterior triangle of the neck.
   c **True.** Although rare, a laryngocoele may be seen in the anterior triangle of the neck. A laryngocoele is an outpouching within the larynx, and is most commonly found in musicians who play wind instruments.
   d **False.** Cervical ribs can be felt in the posterior triangle of the neck.
   e **True.** A cystic hygroma is a swelling of the jugular lymph sac. Cystic hygromas are present in the anterior triangle and may transilluminate. Thyroid masses and thyroglossal and dermoid cysts tend to be found in the midline rather than in the anterior triangle. Lymph nodes may be palpated as lumps in the posterior triangle.

10. a **True.** The tongue is a common site of oral cancers.
    b **False.** The oral cavity is lined by squamous epithelium, so cancers in this region invariably tend to be of squamous origin.
    c **True.** The ulcer-like appearance can mask the sinister nature of these cancers. It is important to take a thorough history of the lesion, and to biopsy it if it has been present for more than 3 weeks.

d **True.** Excessive consumption of alcohol and smoking are important risk factors for oral cancers.

e **True.** Leukoplakia is a white plaque or patch on the inside of the cheeks within the mouth. It may later develop into cancer.

11. a **True.**
    b **True.**
    c **False.** This term does not exist.
    d **True.**
    e **True.**

12. a **True.** In hyperthyroidism the thyroid gland produces excess thyroxine, so the patient's metabolic processes subsequently function excessively.
    b **True.**
    c **True.**
    d **False.** Due to the excess thyroxine produced in hyperthyroidism, the patient may complain of weight loss rather than weight gain.
    e **False.** Patients with hyperthyroidism will have tachycardia and may complain of palpitations.

13. a **True.** This is a characteristic sign of hypothyroidism.
    b **True.**
    c **False.** Diarrhoea is usually associated with hyperthyroidism. Patients with hypothyroidism may complain of constipation.
    d **True.**
    e **True.** Psychiatric manifestations of endocrine conditions are common. Depression may occur in hypothyroid patients.

14. a **True.** One of the complications of a thyroidectomy is damage to the parathyroid glands. These glands are intimately linked to the thyroid gland and are located just behind it. The parathyroid glands are responsible for calcium homeostasis within the body. When removing the thyroid gland it is possible to accidently damage or remove the parathyroid glands as well. As a result, the patient may become hypocalcaemic if they are not given calcium supplementation. The Trousseau sign is elicited by inflating a blood pressure cuff, which results in carpal spasm in hypocalcaemia.
    b **True.** Chvostek's sign is elicited by tapping in the region of the facial nerve, which results in a facial spasm in hypocalcaemia.

c **False.** De Musset's sign is the rhythmic head bobbing that is seen in aortic regurgitation.

d **False.** Pistol-shot femoral pulse sounds are also noted in aortic regurgitation.

e **True.** This characteristic posture is seen in hypocalcaemia.

15. a **False.** In hyperthyroidism there will be a low concentration of TSH, as it is being suppressed by the high levels of T3 and T4.

b **True.** A low TSH level is to be expected in hyperthyroidism, for the above-mentioned reason.

c **True.** The thyroid gland is not reacting to the low TSH level, and is continuing to produce T3 despite the low TSH concentration.

d **False.** T3 is produced by the thyroid gland and so its levels are invariably high in patients with hyperthyroidism.

e **False.** This forms part of the liver function tests, not thyroid function tests. It has no role in the diagnosis of thyroid disease.

16. a **False.** The parathyroid glands produce parathyroid hormone, which acts on the kidneys and results in hypercalcaemia, not hypocalcaemia. It also causes hypophosphataemia and a low urinary calcium level.

b **True.** Primary hyperthyroidism is usually due to a lone adenoma, but may occasionally be due to two or more adenomas.

c **False.** Like most cancers, it is more common in the elderly.

d **False.** It is uncommonly due to cancer, but more commonly due to hyperplasia and benign adenomas.

e **False.** Thyroid-stimulating hormone (TSH) acts on the thyroid gland, not on the parathyroid gland. The parathyroid glands react directly to low calcium levels.

17. a **True.** Other types include follicular, medullary and anaplastic thyroid cancers.

b **False.** Fine-needle aspiration is important in the diagnosis of this cancer, and does not produce 'seeding' of the cancer.

c **False.** Surgery is the main treatment for localised thyroid cancers. Radiation may be used if the cancer appears to be amenable to this. Thyroid cancers are generally not sensitive to, or treated with, chemotherapy.

d **True.** Papillary thyroid cancer has a good prognosis, and 95% of patients survive for more than 5 years.

e **False.** It is three times more common in women, and has a worse prognosis if detected in a male patient.

18. a **False.** It is more common in the elderly.
   b **True.** It is more common in women than in men.
   c **False.** A total thyroidectomy greatly improves the prognosis.
   d **False.** The larger the cancer, the poorer the prognosis.
   e **False.** It is the second commonest thyroid cancer after papillary thyroid cancer.

19. a **True.** Medullary cancer is more common in people in their forties.
   b **True.** Patients who present with medullary cancer should have their parathyroid and adrenal glands investigated to ascertain whether MEN syndrome is present.
   c **False.** Medullary thyroid cancer grows relatively slowly.
   d **True.** Common sites of metastasis for medullary thyroid cancer include bone, brain, lungs and liver.
   e **True.** These range from autosomal-dominant inheritance to the presence of various syndromes, such as MEN syndrome.

20. a **True.** Anaplastic thyroid cancer can arise from any of the differentiated thyroid cancers, not just papillary cancer.
   b **False.** Anaplastic thyroid cancer is a very aggressive, fast-growing and invasive cancer.
   c **False.** Anaplastic thyroid cancer commonly spreads to the lungs and other sites.
   d **False.** Anaplastic thyroid cancer is very difficult to manage. The option of thyroidectomy is often too late for any curative intention, as the cancer has already spread. Chemotherapy and radiotherapy may be used to help to slow the growth of the cancer.
   e **False.** Anaplastic thyroid cancer has an extremely poor prognosis, with patients dying within less than 1 year after diagnosis.

21. a **True.** During a thyroidectomy, the recurrent laryngeal nerve must be visualised and preserved. This nerve innervates the vocal cords. However, occasionally the nerve is unexpectedly damaged or cut, and as a result the patient has a hoarse voice. This may be transient, and recover completely, or it may be permanent. The patient must be made aware of this possibility.
   b **True.** Usually, after the completion of the thyroidectomy, a drainage tube is placed in the wound and attached to a suction machine before the wound is sutured up. However, occasionally the tube may become blocked or dislodged, or a haematoma

may form in any case and begin to compress the trachea. This can quickly lead to respiratory compromise. If a patient is on the ward after a thyroidectomy with respiratory compromise and appears to have a swollen neck, the neck sutures must be cut immediately to open and evacuate the haematoma. This is a life-saving intervention and it should not be delayed. The patient should be advised that they will be under close supervision after the procedure to help to prevent haematoma formation.

c **False.** Epistaxis (bleeding from the nose) is not a complication of a thyroidectomy.

d **True.** The four parathyroid glands responsible for calcium metabolism are located just behind the thyroid gland. During a thyroidectomy it is possible to damage or inadvertently excise these glands. This can result in either transient or permanent hypocalcaemia. The patient should be advised about the possible need for lifelong calcium supplementation.

e **True.** As with all invasive procedures, infection is always a possibility.

22. a **False.** Basal-cell cancers are usually slow-growing. The head and neck are exposed to the sun and are common sites of skin cancer. The main types of skin cancer include melanomas and basal-cell and squamous-cell cancers.

b **True.** Lighter skin has less protection against UV radiation and is therefore more susceptible to UV damage. This damage can accumulate and lead to the development of skin cancer.

c **True.** Basal-cell cancers are the most common type of skin cancer.

d **False.** Although basal-cell cancers are highly infiltrating, they rarely metastasise.

e **False.** Solar keratosis is the premalignant form of squamous-cell cancer. It is not a premalignant form of basal-cell cancer.

23. a **True.** Clark's classification, Breslow thickness and the TNM staging system are all appropriate for melanoma. All of them yield important management and prognostic information.

b **False.** When considering the tight proportions of the facial features, a 5 cm margin will have a devastating cosmetic effect and will be a difficult wound to close. A 10 mm margin is usually sufficient when removing a shallow (1 mm thick) melanoma from the head and neck.

c **True.** See explanation for the first part of this question.

d **True.** Nothing will be achieved by removing the melanoma if some cancerous cells are being harboured in the lymph nodes. A neck dissection involves removing the affected lymph nodes to prevent further spread of the cancer.

e **True.** The risk is greatly increased if a close relative has had melanoma. It is essential to take a thorough family history when diagnosing and managing all head and neck cancers.

24. a **True.** The TNM is a widely accepted cancer staging system, and it is important to understand it when studying head and neck surgery, as it dictates the prognosis.

b **True.** This is staged by scoring on a scale of 0–3.

c **True.** The 'N' staging refers to both the size and number of lymph nodes involved.

d **True.** As described above, 'N' refers to both the size and number of lymph nodes involved. With reference to the head and neck region, a score of 0 indicates that there is no local lymph node involvement. A score of 1 indicates that a local solitary lymph node is involved, and that it is less than 3 cm in size. A score of 2 indicates that either a local solitary lymph node of more than 3 cm, but less than 6 cm in size, is involved, or that multiple ipsilateral or bilateral nodes of any size less than 6 cm are involved. A score of 3 indicates that an involved local lymph node, whether solitary or one of many, is greater than 6 cm in size.

e **False.** 'M' does refer to metastasis, but is only scored on a scale of 0–1, where 0 indicates the absence of metastasis, and 1 indicates its presence.

25. a **True.** The epiglottis is part of the larynx. It closes off the entrance to the larynx and so prevents aspiration of solids and liquids during swallowing.

b **True.** Phonation is the process of converting the flow of air into recognisable sounds. The vocal cords are part of the larynx and are involved in phonation.

c **False.** The larynx is not involved in the sense of smell. The olfactory nerve fibres in the nose are responsible for the sense of smell.

d **True.** There are cough receptors located in the larynx, which stimulate a cough reflex if stimulated by aspirated material.

e **False.** The larynx is not involved in proprioception.

26. a **True.** Sialadenitis is the inflammation of the salivary glands due to infection.

b **True.**

c **True.** The flow of saliva may be prevented due to sialolithiasis (the presence of calculi or stones in the salivary ducts). Static saliva provides a perfect medium for bacterial growth and subsequent infection.

d **False.** It is commonly caused by *Staphylococcus aureus*. However, other bacteria may also be responsible. Listeria meningitis does not cause acute sialadenitis.

e **True.** Gently massaging the salivary gland can improve salivary flow and so alleviate the inflammation. Treatment may also include the use of antibiotics, compression and hydration.

27. **a** **True.** The parotid gland is situated along the zygomatic arch in the region of the cheeks. It produces saliva which enters the mouth via the parotid duct and through an opening next to the second upper molar tooth.

b **False.** The lacrimal gland is situated just above the lateral aspect of the eye, and is responsible for the formation of tears. It does not produce saliva.

c **True.** The sublingual glands are located under the tongue and actively produce saliva to keep the mouth moist.

d **True.** The submandibular gland is located under the mandible just beneath the chin.

e **False.** The pituitary gland is located in the cranium and is responsible for endocrine homeostasis in the body. It does not produce saliva.

28. **a** **False.** They are almost five times more common in the submandibular gland. The reason for this is unclear.

b **True.** Salivary calculi can result in salivary stasis. This forms a breeding ground for bacteria and can result in inflammation of the salivary glands (sialadenitis).

c **True.** This occurs when the calculi obstruct the flow of saliva. During eating, the salivary glands are stimulated and produce large amounts of saliva. As the saliva cannot flow and escape, this causes the gland to swell and results in gland pain.

d **False.** Salivary calculi are made worse by dehydration, as this precipitates the formation of calculi. Thorough hydration should be encouraged.

e **False.** Patients with gout are more likely to develop salivary calculi, and many calculi are composed of uric acid.

29. a **False.** This child is most probably suffering from mumps. Salivary calculi are rare in this age group.

b **False.** Antibiotics are of no help here. Mumps is treated conservatively with fluids and painkillers.

c **True.** The MMR vaccine immunises against mumps. The media controversy regarding this vaccine is unfounded, and the vaccine is a life-saving preventive measure.

d **True.** He is at risk of sensorineural hearing loss, and will require audiometry when he is more stable.

e **True.** Encephalitis may result, which can be fatal.

30. a **True.** Sjögren's syndrome is caused by the formation of autoantibodies which attack the secretory glands of the body.

b **False.** Sjögren's syndrome presents with dry mucous membranes. Patients complain of a dry mouth and eye irritation.

c **True.** Many patients with Sjögren's syndrome benefit from artificial tear drops, which can relieve irritation. Management is supportive, as there is no definitive cure for the disease.

d **False.** These antibody tests will be positive in patients with Sjögren's syndrome. The erythrocyte sedimentation rate (ESR) may also be high.

e **False.** Schirmer's test involves touching the eye with a thin piece of paper and measuring the length of paper that subsequently becomes saturated. This test shows a characteristically reduced length of saturation in individuals with Sjögren's syndrome.

31. a **True.** Parotidectomy can be divided into superficial, deep or total parotidectomy. The facial nerve is at risk in all types of parotidectomy, but the risk is higher in a deep and total parotidectomy than in a superficial one.

b **True.** Frey's syndrome describes gustatory sweating. Following surgery on the parotid gland, various nerve fibres that have been damaged may form abnormal connections, as a result of which salivation can result in sweating.

c **True.** This nerve may be damaged during parotid surgery, resulting in sensory loss around the ear. However, this commonly resolves over time.

d **False.** The vestibulocochlear nerve innervates the inner ear. Parotid surgery does not result in damage to this nerve.

e **True.** Infection is a generic complication that can follow any invasive procedure.

32. a **True.**
    b **True.**
    c **True.**
    d **True.**
    e **False.** This is the natural deterioration of vision with age.

33. a **True.** A total laryngectomy involves removal of the larynx, and speech therapy is essential postoperatively to ensure that the patient can develop the skills and techniques necessary for effective communication.
    b **True.** The scar tissue resulting from laryngeal surgery can narrow parts of the pharynx or oesophagus.
    c **False.** A laryngectomy does not affect hearing.
    d **False.** A total laryngectomy means that the larynx has been totally removed and that the trachea is now totally separate from the pharynx and oesophagus. There is therefore no risk of aspiration.
    e **False.** There is no link between total laryngectomy and chronic sinusitis.

34. a **True.** These nodes mainly drain the scalp.
    b **False.** There are no groups of lymph nodes bearing this name.
    c **True.** These mainly drain the thyroid gland.
    d **True.** These drain the ears and scalp.
    e **True.** These are located deep to the sternocleidomastoid muscle, and drain the other nodes of the neck.

35. a **True.** This involves expelling air through the oesophagus in order to generate speech. The problem is with the relatively short phrases that can be uttered in one go, and the difficulty in learning this technique.
    b **True.** This relies on a technique similar to gastro-oesophageal speech, but the air originates from the lungs and not the stomach. This allows a more natural speech.
    c **True.** Sign language and writing/drawing are all options available to patients. Sign language relies on the recipient also understanding sign language. For this reason it is considered secondary to voice-generating techniques.
    d **True.** These electronic devices generate vibrations in the neck and throat. The vibrations produce sound, and the patients then articulate and modulate these sounds and convert them into words. However, the words produced sound quite robotic.

e **False.** Eye contact will not convey a person's thoughts, and it is not a method of communication (although it may aid communication!).

36. a **True.** Laryngeal cancer can affect any part of the larynx. The larynx is divided into the supraglottis, glottis and subglottis. Laryngeal cancer most commonly affects the glottis, which is the narrowest part of the larynx.
    b **True.** The presence of a hoarse voice is an important observation. The pain caused by laryngeal cancer may be brushed off by the patient as a cold or a sore throat that has not resolved. You should enquire about the systemic oncological symptoms of tiredness and weight loss.
    c **True.** The vast majority of laryngeal cancers are squamous-cell cancers.
    d **False.** Depending on the site and type of cancer, laryngeal cancer can aggressively metastasise to local structures.
    e **True.** Subglottic laryngeal cancers, although more rare, have a higher rate of metastasis, and therefore a poorer prognosis than supraglottic and glottic laryngeal cancers. Laryngeal cancers are graded using the TNM staging system.

37. a **True.** 5-Fluorouracil inhibits the S-phase of the cell cycle and thus prevents cell replication and cancer growth. It is important to be aware of chemotherapy in oncological surgery, as it offers an important alternative to an invasive procedure. It can often be used as a neoadjuvant before surgery, and may thus improve the outcome. Common side-effects of many chemotherapeutic agents include nausea, vomiting, myelosuppression, infections, hair loss and tiredness.
    b **False.** Tramadol is an opiate analgesic and has no effect on cancer growth.
    c **False.** Metronidazole is an antibiotic and has no effect on cancer growth.
    d **True.** This binds to DNA and prevents replication.
    e **True.** Although it is also used as a disease-modifying anti-rheumatic drug (DMARD) in inflammatory rheumatological and gastrointestinal diseases, methotrexate is a potent chemotherapeutic agent.

38. a **True.** Although this question may appear difficult, only basic anatomical knowledge is required to answer it. The question is

asking which structures run alongside the carotid arteries. The sympathetic chain can be damaged or compressed by carotid body tumours, resulting in Horner's syndrome. As the tumour enlarges and compresses the carotid artery and the surrounding nerves, other symptoms may also occur, such as pain, tongue paresis, hoarseness and dysphagia.

b **True.** The hypoglossal nerve can become compressed by carotid body tumours.

c **True.** Tumours can compress and stimulate nerve fibres, resulting in pain.

d **True.** Carotid body tumours can compress the recurrent laryngeal nerve.

e **True.** The carotid tumour can actually be felt as a mass in the anterior triangle.

39. a **False.** Vesicles are found in the auditory canal in Ramsay Hunt syndrome, not in Bell's palsy. Bell's palsy is an idiopathic weakness of the facial nerve that results in drooping and asymmetry of one side of the face. It is named after Sir Charles Bell (1774–1842), a Scottish anatomist, surgeon and physiologist. His name is also given to Bell's phenomenon and Bell's nerve (the long thoracic nerve), which are among his other discoveries.

b **True.** Bell's palsy affects the facial nerve, which is the seventh cranial nerve.

c **True.** The facial nerve innervates the muscles of facial expression. Bell's palsy can present with drooping of the corner of the mouth, with or without forehead sparing. The involvement of the forehead can help to identify whether an upper or lower motor neuron has been affected, as there is forehead sparing if the upper motor neuron is involved. The level of weakness can be graded using either the House–Brackmann scale or Yanagihara's 40-point scoring system.

d **False.** Although Bell's palsy is idiopathic by definition, herpes simplex virus has been implicated as the cause. Epstein–Barr virus has no involvement in Bell's palsy.

e **True.** As described above, Bell's palsy is an idiopathic unilateral facial weakness.

40. a **True.**
b **True.**
c **True.**

d **False.** There is no 'maxillary' branch of the facial nerve. There is a mandibular branch of the facial nerve.

e **True.**

41. a **False.** Sinus cancer can grow to a large size before it causes any symptoms. As a result these cancers, although rare, are usually detected late and have often metastasised by the time of detection.

b **False.** An MRI is the usual radiological modality used for visualisation of the extent of the cancer. A radiograph will only show bone and calcified structures. Sinus cancer is of soft tissue origin, so will not be directly visible on a radiograph.

c **True.** The main symptoms of sinus cancer are due to its space-occupying effect. It can cause nasal obstruction and chronic sinusitis, as well as nosebleeds.

d **True.** The maxillary sinus is most often affected by sinus cancer.

e **True.** The majority of sinus cancers are squamous-cell cancers. They are difficult to treat, and require a multi-disciplinary team consisting not only of head and neck surgeons, but also possibly requiring input from maxillofacial and plastic surgeons. The management plan must be decided by the patient after all of the advantages and disadvantages of the different techniques available have been discussed.

42. a **True.**

b **True.**

c **True.** This sinus is most often affected by sinus cancer.

d **False.** No sinus with this name exists.

e **True.**

43. a **False.** The larynx is a separate entity from the pharynx.

b **True.** The oral pharynx is located posterior to the oral cavity.

c **True.** The laryngopharynx or hypopharynx is located posterior to the larynx.

d **True.** The nasopharynx is located posterior to the nasal cavity.

e **False.** This term does not exist.

44. a **True.**

b **True.**

c **False.**

d **True.**

e **False.**

45. a **True.** However, there are a number of additional minor salivary glands, in the labial, buccal, lingual and palatal mucosa.

b **True.** Salivary secretion is mainly controlled by parasympathetic signals from the superior and inferior salivatory nuclei. Sympathetic stimulation can also increase salivation marginally. The sympathetic nerves originate from the superior cervical ganglia and travel along the surface of blood vessels to the salivary glands.

c **True.** The glossopharyngeal nerve innervates the parotid gland, whereas the facial nerve innervates the sublingual and submandibular glands.

d **True.** The facial nerve traverses the base of the skull, passing through the stylomastoid foramen and then through the parotid gland, where it divides into its five main branches (temporal, zygomatic, buccal, mandibular and cervical).

e **False.** The saliva produced is usually slightly alkaline.

46. a **True.**

b **False.** It usually occurs in elderly, debilitated and dehydrated individuals.

c **True.** Other contributing factors include some drugs (e.g. oral contraceptive pill, thiouracil) and alcohol.

d **True.** Insufficient saliva production can lead to difficulty in swallowing.

e **True.** Infection is often the cause of inflammation.

47. a **True.** This is because the secretions of submandibular glands tend to contain higher levels of calcium.

b **True.**

c **True.**

d **False.** Small stones may spontaneously pass through the duct, and symptoms will subsequently settle. In this case the patient may be treated conservatively with rehydration, painkillers and sialogogues.

e **True.**

48. a **False.** Around 80% of tumours are found in the parotid gland. These are usually benign and slow-growing tumours which may become malignant over a period of years. Only 10% of tumours occur in the submandibular gland.

b **True.**

c **True.**

d **True.** Diagnosis requires fine-needle aspiration biopsy.

e **False.** Around 80% of minor salivary gland tumours are malignant.

49. a **True.** The muscles of mastication (such as the masseter and temporalis muscles) are derived from the first pharyngeal arch.

b **True.** The respective mandibular and maxillary branches of the trigeminal nerve are also embryologically derived from the first pharyngeal arch.

c **True.** The temporalis is a muscle of mastication and so is derived from the first pharyngeal arch.

d **True.**

e **False.** The muscles of facial expression (such as the orbicularis oris muscle) are derived from the second pharyngeal arch.

50. a **True.** A higher incidence of buccal carcinoma is found in southern Asia. Once treated, these cancers have a high likelihood of reoccurrence.

b **True.** Alcohol and tobacco consumption are well-known risk factors for buccal carcinoma.

c **True.** Surgery has an important role, but radiotherapy and chemotherapy are equally important factors in the management of this difficult cancer.

d **False.** Although Epstein–Barr virus is linked to nasopharyngeal cancer, there is no known association between the virus and buccal carcinoma.

e **True.** In the vast majority of cases, buccal carcinoma is of squamous-cell origin.

51. a **False.** Oral tongue cancer is most commonly of squamous-cell origin.

b **True.** The tongue has an important role in the fine manipulation of sounds essential for speech. Surgical excision of an oral tongue cancer can have a significant impact on a person's voice.

c **False.** Smoking is a risk factor for the development of cancer of the tongue.

d **False.** A gastrectomy is the term used to describe the removal of the stomach. A glossectomy (removal of the tongue) can be used to treat severe oral tongue cancer.

e **True.** The tongue is important in the swallowing process, and oral tongue cancer can be severe enough to affect swallowing.

52. a **False.** The platysma is the first muscle to be incised during a neck dissection, but it is not excised.

b **False.** Unintentionally cutting the common carotid artery can have disastrous consequences.

c **True.** The omohyoid muscle is excised during this procedure.

d **False.** It is very important to visualise and preserve the vagus nerve.

e **False.** The phrenic nerve is identified and preserved during this procedure.

53. a **True.** The ansa cervicalis is part of the cervical plexus. It supplies the sternothyroid, sternohyoid and omohyoid, and contributes innervations to the geniohyoid.

b **True.**

c **False.** The pectoralis major and minor are innervated by the medial and lateral pectoral nerves.

d **False.** The sternocleidomastoid is innervated by the accessory nerve.

e **True.**

54. a **True.** Part of the innervation of the middle ear is via the glossopharyngeal and vagus nerves. Therefore a small hidden throat or tongue-base tumour may present first as a unilateral otalgia.

b **False.** A patient with a persistent change in voice should be referred to an ENT surgeon for a thorough ENT examination, and direct visualisation of the larynx.

c **False.** Incisional or excisional biopsies of neck lumps should be avoided, as they can compromise further treatment and prognosis. A fine-needle aspiration biopsy is the first investigation of choice. Patients with neck lumps should be referred initially to a head and neck surgeon (ENT or maxillofacial surgeon).

d **True.**

e **False.** Lymphoma is only one of many possible causes of a neck lump. It is therefore preferable to obtain a fine-needle biopsy diagnosis first before exposing the patient to what may be unnecessary radiation.

Index